# Advanced Endodontics

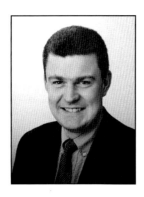

John S Rhodes qualified from King's College London in 1990, where he was awarded the Claudius Ash prize in conservation and the Jose Souyave endodontic prize. He continued his postgraduate education at Guy's Hospital London, where he achieved a distinction in the Endodontic MSc. He is registered on the GDC specialist list in endodontics and now runs a busy endodontic referral practice in Poole, Dorset.

John S Rhodes lectures widely in the UK and provides numerous postgraduate endodontic courses. He has published research papers in several refereed journals and is co-author of the endodontic textbook *Endodontics: Problem-Solving in Clinical Practice.*

# Advanced Endodontics
## Clinical Retreatment and Surgery

John S Rhodes BDS(LOND) MSC MFGDP(UK) MRD RCS(ED)
*Specialist in endodontics*
The Endodontic Practice
Poole, UK

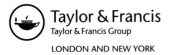
Taylor & Francis
Taylor & Francis Group

LONDON AND NEW YORK

© 2006 Taylor & Francis, an imprint of the Taylor & Francis Group
Taylor & Francis Group is the Academic Division of Informa plc

First published in the United Kingdom in 2006 by Taylor & Francis, an imprint of the Taylor & Francis Group, 2 Park Square, Milton Park, Abingdon, Oxon OX14 4RN

Tel:          +44 (0)20 7017 6000
Fax:          +44 (0)20 7017 6699
E-mail:       info.medicine@tandf.co.uk
Website:      www.tandf.co.uk/medicine

Although every effort has been made to ensure that all owners of copyright material have been acknowledged in this publication, we would be glad to acknowledge in subsequent reprints or editions any omissions brought to our attention.

Although every effort has been made to ensure that drug doses and other information are presented accurately in this publication, the ultimate responsibility rests with the prescribing physician. Neither the publishers nor the authors can be held responsible for errors or for any consequences arising from the use of information contained herein. For detailed prescribing information or instructions on the use of any product or procedure discussed herein, please consult the prescribing information or instructional material issued by the manufacturer.

A CIP record for this book is available from the British Library.

Library of Congress Cataloging-in-Publication Data
Data available on application

ISBN 1-84184-436-5
ISBN 978-1-84184-436-7

Distributed in the United States and Canada by
Thieme New York
333 Seventh Avenue
New York, NY 10001

Distributed in the rest of the world by
Thomson Publishing Services
Cheriton House
North Way
Andover
Hampshire SP10 5BE, UK
Tel:          +44 (0)1264 332424
E-mail:       salesorder.tandf@thomsonpublishingservices.co.uk

Composition by Newgen Imaging Systems (P) Ltd, Chennai, India

Printed and bound in Great Britain by CPI, Bath

# CONTENTS

# ACKNOWLEDGEMENTS

I wish to thank the following for kind permission to reproduce figures:
Dr CP Sproat: Figure 8:15
Dr J Aquilina: Figures 6:18 and 6:19
Mr DA Oultram (Optident UK): Figures 7:09, 7:10
Mr S Bonsor, Mr G Pearson and Mr J Williams: Figures 7:11, 7:12, 7:13

I would like to acknowledge the contributions of the following people and companies who provided equipment for photography: Neil Conduit of QED, Douglas Pitman of DP Medical, David Mason of J&S Davis, Dentsply UK, Henry Schien UK, Optident and Denfotex; the staff at *The Endodontic Practice* who agreed to be photographed for illustrative material; my parents, who helped edit the many drafts; and my wife Sarah and family, who supported me patiently while I compiled this book.

# PREFACE

This book is intended for the general practitioner with a special interest in endodontics, students undergoing specialist training and specialists alike.

Endodontic retreatment poses many practical challenges. Advances in scientific knowledge and the integration of operating microscopes into endodontic practice have seen the possibilities for predictable endodontic treatment and retreatment expand dramatically.

*Advanced Endodontics: Clinical Retreatment and Surgery* describes many of the techniques and methods available for practitioners who wish to undertake the planning and treatment of complex endodontic retreatment.

The pages are copiously illustrated with high-quality photographs and case reports which are used to demonstrate practical non-surgical and surgical techniques. The text is referenced to provide a comprehensive but discreet source of scientific evidence, principles and further reading.

Knowledge and theory are important in managing complex endodontic retreatment cases, but cannot be a substitute for essential practical and clinical experience. These skills need to be learned and practiced. Novices should always start with the simplest cases and never proceed beyond their confidence or skill level. Numerous practical courses are available for instruction on retreatment techniques and attendance on them can only be encouraged.

John S Rhodes

# DEDICATION

This book is dedicated to my endodontic mentors:

Professor Tom Pitt Ford

and

Dr Chris Stock

# 1 RATIONALE FOR ENDODONTIC RETREATMENT

## INTRODUCTION

Patients increasingly expect to retain their natural dentition and are often reluctant to have teeth extracted. Endodontic retreatment or surgery may offer the patient a second chance to save a root-treated tooth that would otherwise be destined for extraction.

The success rate for root canal treatment carried out with currently accepted principles should be high. Indeed, published figures of between 70 and 95% have been quoted in studies using samples derived from teaching hospitals.[1] However, there is marked variation in the ability of operators to achieve successful results. Some studies using data collected from general practice have shown relatively low success rates for root canal treatment. An assessment into the standard of root canal treatment in England and Wales for example, showed that 97% of molar root canal treatment and 84% of canine and incisor root canal treatment had technical difficulties,[2] whereas in Scotland over 58% of root filled teeth showed signs of periapical radiolucency.[3] Similar radiographic results have been found in studies from the USA[4] and Holland.[5] The prevalence of endodontically treated teeth showing periradicular radiolucency in Scandinavia has consistently been reported to be between 25 and 35%.[6] Obviously, there is a contradiction between what is achievable and what is actually achieved. So why does primary endodontic treatment fail?

Endodontic failure comprises:

- biological failings (infection)
- cysts
- root fracture
- incorrect diagnosis and primary treatment
- foreign body reactions
- healing with scar
- neuropathic problems
- economic constraints.

## BIOLOGICAL FAILINGS

The most common reason for failure of root treatment is microbial infection. Microorganisms and their byproducts have been isolated from the root canal system and the external surface of the root in failed cases. They may have persisted following a previous attempt at root canal treatment or gained access through coronal microleakage.

### Intraradicular Infection

It is well documented in clinical studies that teeth with technically deficient root fillings are more likely to be associated with periapical radiolucencies. If a root filling is of poor quality, the root canal system may not have been effectively disinfected or could have become reinfected through coronal microleakage (Figures 1.1, 1.2). The apical portion of the root canal system can contain bacteria and necrotic tissue

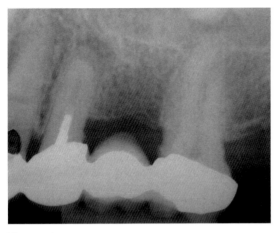

**Figure 1.1**

This radiograph shows a chronic periapical lesion associated with the maxillary left first premolar. The tooth has been restored with a post and core and is an abutment for a bridge. There is little root filling material present and the root canal would undoubtedly be infected.

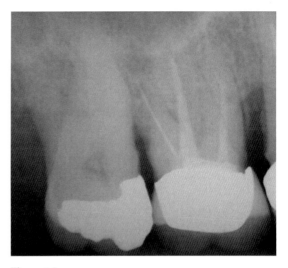

**Figure 1.2**

In this case the maxillary right first molar has been root filled. The root filling material is short in the mesiobuccal and palatal roots but there is little evidence of periapical pathology. The distobuccal canal has a fractured stainless steel instrument in it. The root canal must be infected, as there is a periapical radiolucency present. The root canal system may have become reinfected by coronal microleakage following root canal treatment because the file provided a poor seal. Alternatively, infected material may not have been removed or could have been carried along the entire length of the root canal prior to the instrument failing. Sufficient numbers of bacteria are now present to cause persistence of the lesion.

substrate even following chemomechanical preparation.[7,8] If the resultant microbial ecosystem is amenable to bacterial survival, a lesion may not heal and root canal treatment would be deemed to have failed (Figure 1.3).

The radiographic appearance of a root canal filling does not give an indication of biological status and, consequently, a satisfactory radiographic result could be failing biologically.[9] A clinical example would be the misuse of carrier-based obturating materials where the canal system may appear to have been well obturated radiographically, but has not been adequately instrumented or disinfected. Usually, all that remains in the canal is the radio-opaque plastic carrier. Root canal retreatment in this instance should have a good chance of success as the failure is basically technical and a good aseptic technique has not been used (Figures 1.4, 1.5).

Rather more complex and difficult to treat would be a situation in which an excellent aseptic technique and high standard of skill has been achieved but the case has failed (Figures 1.6, 1.7).

If the root canal filling fails to provide a complete seal, seepage of tissue fluids could theoretically provide a substrate for

bacterial growth. Studies have reported the occurrence of viable bacteria in root-treated teeth with persistent periradicular lesions.[10,11] To be viable in such conditions, the bacteria have to survive periods of starvation or nutrient depletion. Bacterial regulatory systems under the control of determined genes are automatically transcribed under adverse conditions. For instance, under conditions of nitrogen starvation, some bacteria are able to scavenge minute traces of ammonia as a nitrogen source. Facultative bacteria may be able to activate alternative metabolic pathways and survive in low concentrations of molecular oxygen by switching from aerobic to anaerobic respiration. Under low concentrations of glucose, some bacteria can activate genes that induce enzyme synthesis to allow the utilization of various alternative organic carbon sources.

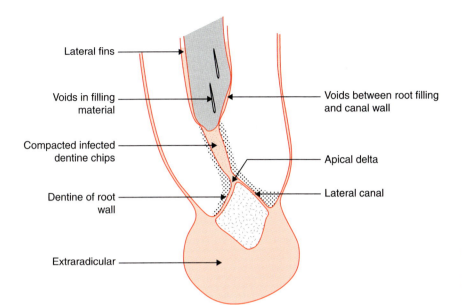

Lateral fins

Voids in filling material

Compacted infected dentine chips

Dentine of root wall

Extraradicular

Voids between root filling and canal wall

Apical delta

Lateral canal

**Figure 1.3**

Potential sites of microbial infection in the failed root-filled tooth.

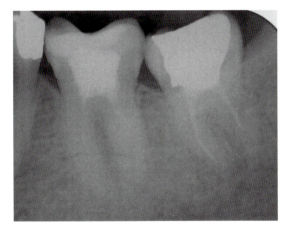

**Figure 1.4**

A Thermafil root filling has been placed in this mandibular second molar. The filling is short in the distal canal, but the mesial canals look reasonably well obturated. A tell-tale sign on the radiograph that this is not the case is 'bunching' of gutta percha in the access cavity. The obturating material has been stripped off the carrier as it was inserted. Only the carrier remains in the root canal.

The availability of nutrients within the root canal system and the ability to survive in a more hostile environment dictate whether the remaining microorganisms will die or remain viable.

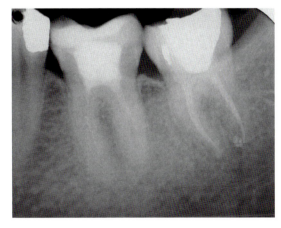

**Figure 1.5**

The previous case retreated. The distal canal has been renegotiated and instrumented. All the canals have been obturated using gutta percha and sealer.

Bacterial infection is the major cause of persistent periapical inflammation following root canal treatment. However, there are technical failings that may predispose the root canal system to inadequate disinfection:

• poor aseptic technique
• incorrect irrigant

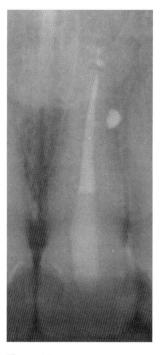

**Figure 1.6**

The root canal of this maxillary left central incisor would appear to have been shaped and disinfected adequately. A lateral canal has subsequently been obturated. The tooth was unfortunately still symptomatic following root canal treatment and there was tenderness over the apex. Root canal retreatment in this instance is going to be complex as the previous attempt is good.

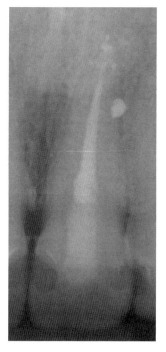

**Figure 1.7**

Root canal retreatment completed. Following removal of the existing root filling material and disinfection, considerably more complex anatomy has been cleaned and obturated in the apical region. It was not possible to remove extruded material from beyond the terminus of the lateral canal.

- inability to prepare the canal to length
- missed canals
- procedural errors
- poor obturation
- poor restoration and coronal microleakage
- resistant bacteria.

### Poor Aseptic Technique

Surveys carried out amongst general dental practitioners show that the majority of root canal treatment is carried out without a rubber dam.[12,13] Practitioners that do not use a rubber dam concomitantly tend not to use biologically active irrigants. The combined effect could have a significant bearing on the likelihood of success, but to date there are no published data proving that the use of a rubber dam increases success rates.

The use of a rubber dam is considered mandatory for root canal treatment by dental teachers and endodontic specialists for many good reasons.

The benefits of using a rubber dam for root canal treatment include:

- prevention of microbial contamination
- the safe use of sodium hypochlorite
- airway protection
- retraction of the soft tissues
- unimpeded vision, which is useful with magnification
- quicker and more pleasant treatment
- reduction of microbial aerosol
- allows the operative field to be dried.

## Incorrect Irrigants

The modern rationale for root canal treatment involves a chemomechanical approach. Bacteria are removed mechanically with instruments but also killed using irrigants which penetrate the complex internal anatomy of the root canal system (Figures 1.8, 1.9).

The primary irrigant in endodontic treatment should have both proteolytic and bacterial killing properties. In this respect, a solution of at least 1% sodium hypochlorite solution is recommended.[14]

Irrigants such as chlorhexidine and iodine in potassium iodide have also been advocated as adjuncts to sodium hypochlorite. Both have antibacterial properties but do not aid the dissolution of organic material. Irrigants such as local anaesthetic or saline have no biologically active properties and will not aid the dissolution of organic material or killing of bacteria. Irrigant choice has a minimal effect on root canal treatment outcome when analysed statistically.

## Inability to Prepare to Length

Failure to achieve patency during preparation can result in inadequate penetration of irrigants. This could result in persistent infection and endodontic failure. The apical 3 mm of a root canal contains the highest percentage of lateral canals and deltas. There is an argument that if mechanical preparation, and consequently irrigant penetration, are 2–3 mm short of the constriction, the hypothetical length of canal that has not been disinfected could be as great as 6–7 mm (Figure 1.10).

Outdated filing techniques such as the stepback method[15] can be fraught with instrumentation errors. Zips and elbows are not uncommon, as stiff stainless steel files used in a linear fashion tend to straighten the canals (Figure 1.11).

These in turn are easily blocked with dentine chips that could potentially be infected. Modern preparation techniques and rotary nickel–titanium instruments are used with a crown-down approach.[16,17] The coronal aspect of the canal is prepared first, allowing much better access to the apical part. The development of nickel–titanium files with tapers greater than standard hand files has eliminated the need to step back. This speeds up preparation and reduces the number of instruments that are required. These developments have improved the

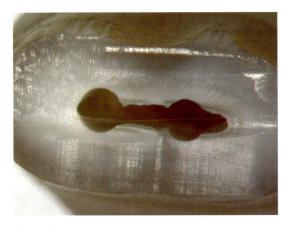

**Figure 1.8**

This is a cross-section of a root canal that has been mechanically prepared using nickel–titanium rotary instruments. It is quite obvious where material has been removed. The areas that are untouched by the files will have to be cleaned using irrigants and medicaments.

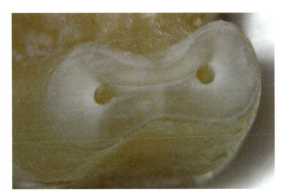

**Figure 1.9**

Nickel–titanium rotary instruments have been used to prepare the mesial root canals of a mandibular molar. The majority of the root canal in this instance has been machined mechanically and therefore some cleaning will have occurred during this process. It is not uncommon to find an isthmus joining the two canals in the apical third of the mesial root of mandibular molars. This would obviously have to be cleaned using irrigants and medicaments.

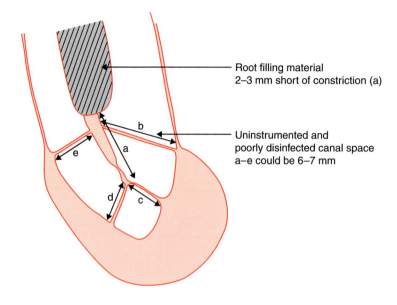

Root filling material
2–3 mm short of constriction (a)

Uninstrumented and
poorly disinfected canal space
a–e could be 6–7 mm

**Figure 1.10**

Inability to prepare to length.

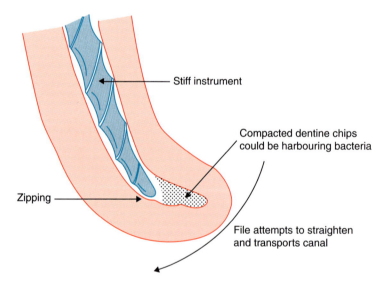

Stiff instrument

Compacted dentine chips
could be harbouring bacteria

Zipping

File attempts to straighten
and transports canal

**Figure 1.11**

File attempts to straighten and transports
canal.

ability to prepare canal systems predictably, while preventing blockage.

## Missed Canals

A missed canal could harbour persistent bacteria. Aberrant or unusual anatomy must therefore be considered in retreatment cases. If a root-filled tooth appears satisfactory from a radiographic perspective but is still symptomatic, a missed canal could be suspected. Maxillary first molars contain two canals in the mesiobuccal root in approximately 78% of teeth.[18] Mandibular incisors have two canals in over 40% of cases[19] and mandibular first molars frequently contain four canals. The clinician must be aware of normal root canal anatomy before re-entering a root canal-treated tooth and be prepared for added complexity in retreatment cases (Figures 1.12–1.14).[20]

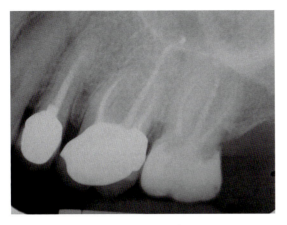

**Figure 1.12**

The maxillary left second molar was root treated and the final result was reasonable. Careful analysis of the radiograph shows that there is likely to be a second mesiobuccal canal that has not been prepared. The tooth was still symptomatic.

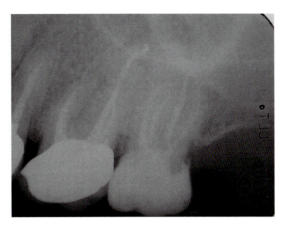

**Figure 1.14**

The second mesiobuccal canal is indeed a separate entity and has been shaped, cleaned and obturated.

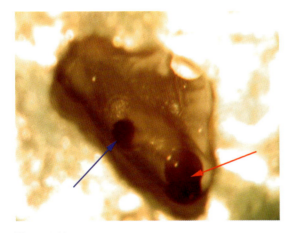

**Figure 1.13**

Under microscopic magnification, a view of the pulp floor reveals the position of a second mesiobuccal canal (indicated by a blue arrow).

## Procedural Errors

Procedural errors occurring during primary root canal treatment of an infected tooth may predispose the treatment to failure by making it more difficult to effectively disinfect the entire root canal system.[21] Inadequate disinfection may therefore reduce the prognosis of initial root treatment and procedural errors decrease the chance of successful retreatment if necessitated.

Ledges are effectively an internal transportation of the canal and can be caused by a file working against compacted dentine chips. This infected material may harbour bacteria that could result in persistent inflammation (Figure 1.15).

Another problem often encountered in retreatment cases is apical transportation. Canals exhibiting apical transportation tend to be under-filled. There may be voids between the filling material and the canal walls in which bacteria could persist. Perforations can result in endodontic failure when they become infected or allow microleakage.[22] In the above situations conventional retreatment is normally recommended, as the principal aim is to eliminate bacteria and related irritants from the root canal system (Figures 1.16–1.18).[23]

## Poor Obturation

The aim of obturation and restoration of the endodontically treated tooth is to achieve a complete seal from the apex to the oral cavity. This prevents the ingress of bacteria by coronal leakage or the persistence of bacterial colonies bathed in nutrients from tissue fluid

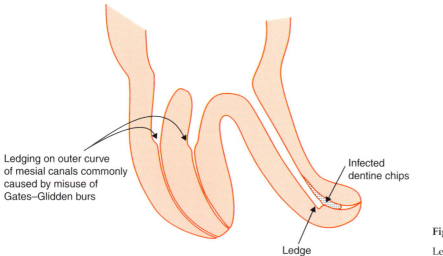

Ledging on outer curve of mesial canals commonly caused by misuse of Gates–Glidden burs

Infected dentine chips

Ledge

**Figure 1.15**

Ledges.

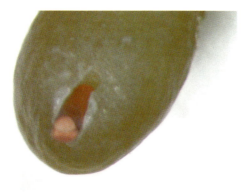

**Figure 1.16**

Apical transportation can occur when the root canal is over-prepared. In this case the palatal root canal of a maxillary molar has been over-prepared with nickel–titanium rotary instruments. Constantly passing the instrument beyond the apical constriction has resulted in straightening of the terminal part of the root canal and a tear adjacent to the gutta percha.

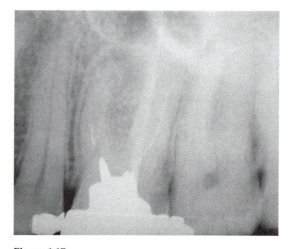

**Figure 1.17**

There are often many obstacles for the clinician to overcome in order to achieve adequate disinfection of the root canal system. In this case the maxillary first molar has fractured instruments in both mesiobuccal and distobuccal canals. The material in the mesiobuccal canal will be more complicated to retrieve than the distobuccal canal. It should be relatively simple to remove compacted gutta percha from the palatal canal.

in the apical region. Modern obturation techniques using thermoplasticized gutta percha aim to obliterate more of the complex root canal system than single cone or silver point techniques, which are now considered obsolete (Figures 1.19–1.21).

It has been claimed that the success rate of root canal treatment is decreased in cases of over-filling.[24] Initially, the toxicity of root canal filling material was considered to be important in this respect,[25] but most of the materials used in root canal obturation are either biocompatible or only show cytotoxicity while

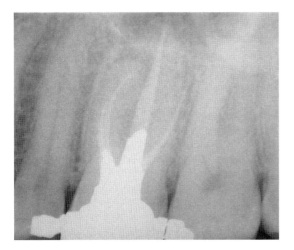

**Figure 1.18**

Root canal retreatment completed. All the separated fragments of instrument were successfully removed. The canals were located, renegotiated, shaped, cleaned and obturated with gutta percha and sealer. An adhesive Nayyar core has been constructed in amalgam. The mesiobuccal root has two separate canals that join in the apical third.

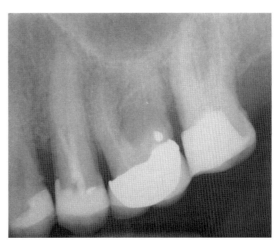

**Figure 1.19**

In this case, the root canals of the maxillary second premolar and first and second molars have been under-prepared and under-filled. In most canals a single cone obturation technique has been utilized. Despite this, it is interesting to note that there is virtually no indication of periapical pathology. Perhaps the root canal treatment was carried out while the teeth were still vital and the root canals were not infected. The restorations on these teeth are destined for replacement and it is therefore necessary to carry out root canal retreatment. In this instance, because of the lack of periapical pathology and obvious technical failings of the previous treatment, a good prognosis should be expected. The distobuccal root of the maxillary left first molar has been resected and an amalgam root end filling placed. The root tip is still present and just visible on the radiograph. The root canal will obviously need to be sealed with conventional restorative material to prevent coronal leakage.

setting.[26] Paraformaldehyde-containing materials, however, are considered to be significantly cytotoxic. It is highly improbable that most of the contemporary endodontic materials are able to induce inflammation in the absence of a concomitant endodontic infection. This is probably why a high success rate can be achieved for root canal treatment in teeth without periapical lesions even in cases of over-filling.[27,28] Infection is the most likely cause of failure when root canals are over-filled, and therefore emphasis on the need to prevent and control endodontic infection efficiently is paramount. Often the apical seal is inadequate in over-filled root canals. Percolation of tissue fluids could provide nutrients for residual microorganisms to proliferate and reach sufficient numbers to induce or perpetuate inflammation. Over-instrumentation often precedes over-filling and in teeth with infected necrotic pulps this causes displacement of infected dentine or debris into the periradicular tissues. In this situation, microorganisms are physically protected from the host defence mechanisms and can sometimes survive extraradicularly.

The presence of infected dentine or cementum chips in the periradicular lesion has been associated with impaired healing (Figures 1.22, 1.23).[29]

## Poor Coronal Restoration

It would appear that the coronal seal could have an important bearing on the success of root-filled teeth.[30] Having thoroughly cleaned the root canal system, the coronal restoration helps to prevent ingress of bacteria into the internal environment and assists in providing a total seal. Good root canal treatment with good coronal restoration achieves the best

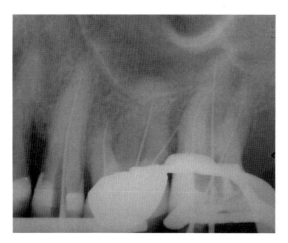

**Figure 1.20**

Filling material has been removed from the three teeth and a diagnostic working length radiograph shows the canals have been successfully renegotiated. Patency has been achieved in all of them.

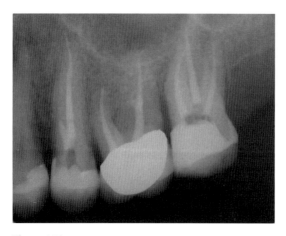

**Figure 1.21**

The case has been obturated using a vertically compacted gutta percha technique. The finished preparations are adequately tapered and the root canal space well sealed with compacted gutta percha and sealer.

outcome, whereas poor root canal treatment and a poor coronal seal may lead to failure.[31,32] Root canals that are well prepared and filled may be able to resist bacterial penetration even upon frank and long-standing exposure for longer than anticipated. A recent study

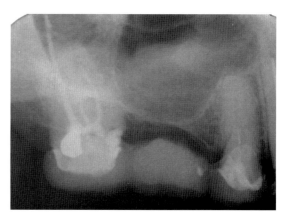

**Figure 1.22**

Root canal treatment has been attempted on both abutments of this three-unit bridge. The mesial abutment shows fractured instruments in the coronal part of the root canal, which should be relatively simple to remove during root canal retreatment. The distal abutment shows a grossly over-extended root filling in the palatal root canal with associated periapical radiolucency. The buccal canals are under-prepared and under-filled. It is likely that the palatal root canal was over-prepared and that infected material has been carried through the apex into the periapical tissues. Root canal retreatment should be perfectly feasible but it is sometimes technically challenging to retrieve over-extended filling materials and there is always the possibility of persistent extraradicular bacteria.

showed no discernible periapical pathology in the majority of 39 roots of 32 teeth exposed to caries or the oral environment for over 3 months. Indeed, some root fillings had been without restoration for several years.[33]

The quality of the coronal seal should however be addressed, as leaking restorations and recurrent caries may compromise the effectiveness of cleaning and shaping by allowing microleakage.[34] It is also important to achieve an effective seal with a rubber dam to prevent salivary contamination and reinfection during root canal preparation (Figures 1.24–1.29).

## Resistant Bacteria

The microbiological flora in failing root-treated teeth has been considered to be different from that of an untreated canal.[35,36] Untreated

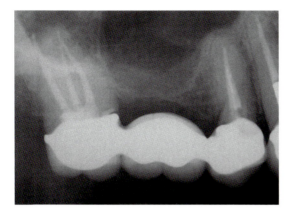

**Figure 1.23**

Retreatment of the previous case. The fractured instruments were simply removed from the mesial abutment under microscopic magnification and the root canals retreated. In the distal abutment the buccal canals have been correctly shaped and now have a tapered form. Over-extended material in the palatal canal has been retrieved and the palatal canal re-prepared and disinfected. All the canals in the distal abutment have been obturated using a vertically compacted gutta percha technique and the case now appears to be adequately sealed.

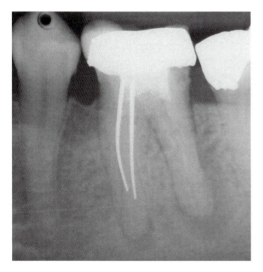

**Figure 1.24**

The coronal restoration in this mandibular left first molar is leaking as a result of caries under the distal margin. There is little root filling material in the distal canal and a large periapical area can be seen around it. The mesial canals have been obturated using a silver point technique and there is also a periapical radiolucency present. The coronal restoration is leaking and will need to be removed prior to root canal retreatment.

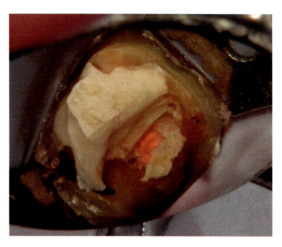

**Figure 1.25**

The crown was simply elevated using a Couplands chisel and the core material dismantled. The superficial layers were removed using a tungsten carbide bur.

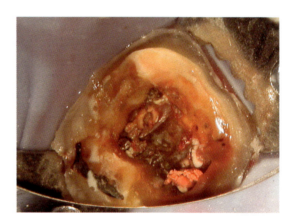

**Figure 1.26**

The remaining material was removed with ultrasonics and this revealed carious dentine and a very messy pulp floor. There had been considerable coronal leakage.

infected canals usually contain a mixed infection in which Gram-negative anaerobic rods predominate. Data from culture-based studies indicate that failed root-treated canals may only have 1–2 species of generally Gram-positive bacteria. It is worth noting that it is extremely challenging to successfully culture bacteria taken from canals during root canal retreatment. In a study by Sundqvist et al, *Enterococcus*

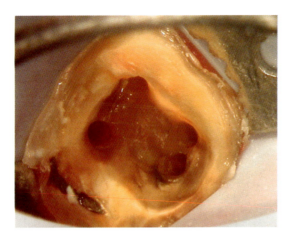

**Figure 1.27**

Carious dentine was removed and the root canals reshaped and disinfected.

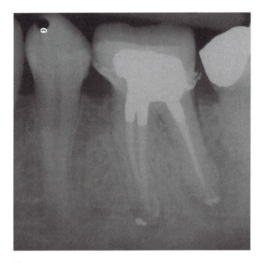

**Figure 1.28**

A postoperative radiograph of the tooth showed the root canals obturated with a vertically compacted gutta percha technique and the coronal substance sealed with an adhesive Nayyar core and temporary acrylic crown.

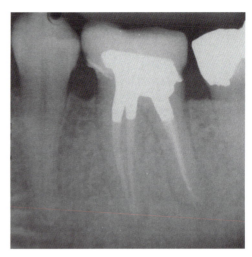

**Figure 1.29**

Six months postoperatively there was good evidence of bony healing and the prognosis for successful root canal retreatment looks high.

*faecalis* was isolated in 38% of failing canals. Increased proportions of *E. faecalis* in teeth lacking adequate seal during treatment have been reported,[34] supporting the suggestion that *E. faecalis* enters the canal during treatment. Strains of *E. faecalis* have shown resistance to intracanal medicaments such as calcium hydroxide and may be present as a monoinfection. More recently, DNA-based identification

techniques have revealed the presence of bacteria in the canals of root-filled teeth with periapical pathology that are rarely revealed in culture studies and have a much greater biodiversity than previously thought.[37]

Yeast-like microorganisms have also been isolated from teeth with failing root fillings[38] which suggests that they may be therapy-resistant. *Candida* species have been shown to be resistant to the most commonly deployed intracanal medicaments in some instances.[39] Therefore, the microflora associated with failing endodontically treated teeth may be extremely resistant and difficult to eradicate during retreatment. Alternative intracanal medicaments and irrigants may be required to enhance the elimination of resistant bacteria in previously root-treated canals. Inadequate primary treatment may therefore have a negative effect on the prognosis of retreatment.

## Extraradicular Infection

It has been suggested that bacterial colonies on the external root surface may be associated with failure. Typically, failure occurs in these cases despite a high standard of primary endodontic treatment. Bacteria such as *Actinomyces israelii* and *Propionibacterium propionicum* have been isolated from such infections.[40–43] Bacterial colonies arranged in biofilms can evade host defences and antimicrobial agents more effectively than planktonic cells. A biofilm can be defined as a microbial population that is attached to an organic or inorganic substrate and surrounded by microbial extracellular products forming an intermicrobial matrix.[44] Bacterial biofilms adjacent to the apical foramen and bacterial colonies located inside periapical granulomas have been reported in teeth that have not responded to root canal treatment.[45] Extraradicular colonies of bacteria are not eradicated by conventional disinfection regimes and therefore, a surgical approach in combination with conventional root canal treatment is often required. It is important to note that when considering retreatment of such a case, conventional disinfection of the root canal is usually indicated as an initial approach prior to surgery. Periradicular biofilms only occur in a small proportion of cases[46] and are consequently only responsible for a low percentage of failed cases. The placement of endodontic medicaments into the periradicular tissues in order to eliminate microorganisms and to decompose periradicular biofilms is not to be recommended. This is because most are cytotoxic and the antimicrobial effects can also be neutralized by tissue fluid.

## CYSTS

The differential diagnosis of a periapical lesion that is greater than 1 cm in diameter with well-defined margins will include the possibility of a radicular cyst.

Radicular cysts are categorized as:

- *apical pocket cysts*, in which the epithelial-lined sac is in communication with the root canal system of the tooth (Figures 1.30, 1.31)
- *apical true cysts*, in which the lesion is completely enclosed by the epithelial lining and has no communication with the root canal system of the tooth (Figure 1.32).

As the pocket cyst is in communication with the root canal, healing should occur in most cases following thorough non-surgical root canal treatment.[47] A true cyst is self-sustaining and

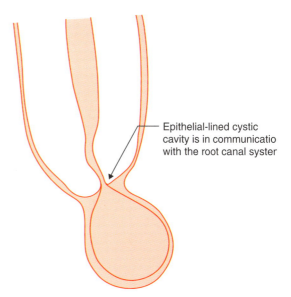

Epithelial-lined cystic cavity is in communicatio with the root canal syster

**Figure 1.30**

Apical pocket cyst.

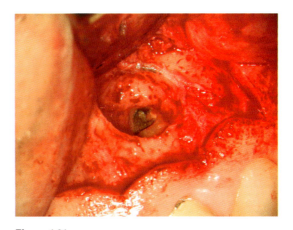

**Figure 1.31**

A radicular cyst was located at the apex of this maxillary central incisor. It may well have been a pocket cyst, as the root tip was located within the tissue lining.

will therefore be unlikely to resolve. In this case, a surgical approach would be required. It is important to note that when considering retreatment of such a case, conventional disinfection of the root canal is normally indicated as an initial approach prior to surgery.

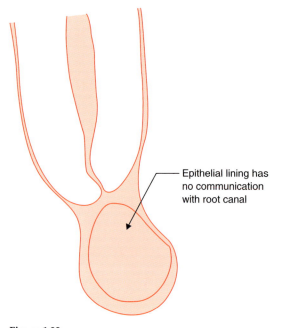

Epithelial lining has
no communication
with root canal

**Figure 1.32**

Apical true cyst.

## CRACKED TEETH AND FRACTURES

There is a difference between a cracked tooth and a vertically fractured tooth. The latter involves movement of the two or more fragments and radiological signs of bone loss associated with the root defect. The long-term prognosis for repair of fractured teeth is poor and extraction is usually the only treatment option.

Careful assessment of the tooth using an operating microscope or loupes and an indicator dye help the clinician evaluate the degree of severity before embarking on root canal retreatment.

Treatment will depend on the severity of the crack. If exposed to the oral cavity, a crack will undoubtedly contain bacteria, which may lead to reinfection of the root-filled canal or inflammation alongside the fracture line in the periodontal ligament.

Cracks that run across the pulp chamber floor may have become infected with bacteria and are therefore more difficult for the clinician to manage. Some teeth will not be

saveable. In others, it may be possible to seal the pulp floor and place a cusp coverage restoration to prolong the life of a tooth for several years.

Teeth requiring endodontic treatment may benefit from the placement of a band to prevent fracture. Following root canal treatment a full coverage crown or cusp coverage restoration is normally recommended to protect the tooth from subsequent fracture (Figures 1.33–1.44).

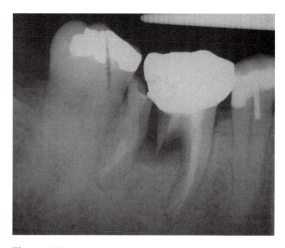

**Figure 1.33**

This root-filled tooth has unfortunately failed as a result of vertical root fracture.

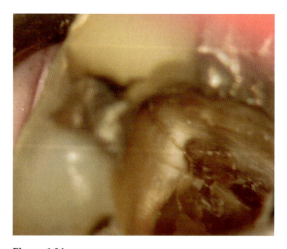

**Figure 1.34**

Good illumination and magnification are essential in order to highlight cracks in teeth. This tooth had a microcrack running down the buccal wall and extending into one of the mesial root canals. Sometimes cracks can be highlighted by staining.

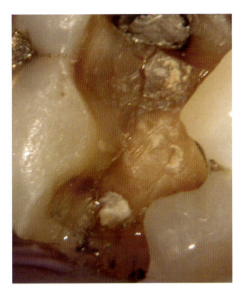

**Figure 1.35**

A serious crack running from the mesial to distal of this mandibular molar has unfortunately resulted in vertical root fracture. The tooth will not be saveable.

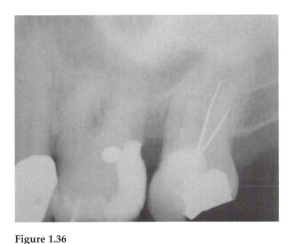

**Figure 1.36**

The maxillary second molar requires root canal retreatment. It has been root filled using a silver point technique. Both points are very short of the root apices and the mesiobuccal canal has not been prepared, cleaned or obturated.

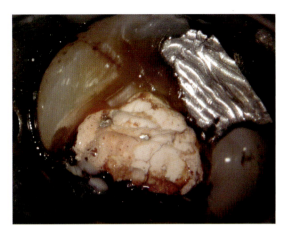

**Figure 1.37**

The superficial core material was removed using a diamond bur to reveal the heads of the silver points.

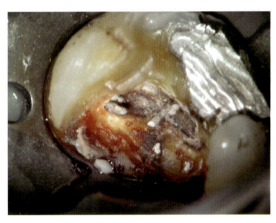

**Figure 1.38**

The remaining core material was then removed with ultrasonics, which left the silver points intact so they could be grasped with Stieglitz forceps and gently removed.

## INCORRECT DIAGNOSIS AND TREATMENT

Diagnosis should follow a methodical and logical progression. Special tests should be applied to ascertain whether or not a pulp is necrotic. Haste in attaining a diagnosis can lead to treatment of the 'wrong tooth' (Figures 1.45–1.47).

## FOREIGN BODY REACTIONS

Rarely, failure may occur because of non-microbial factors. Foreign body reactions against cholesterol crystals derived from

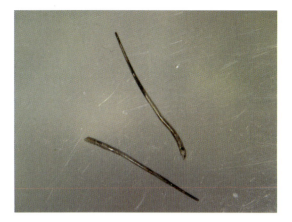

**Figure 1.39**

The silver point root fillings are removed intact.

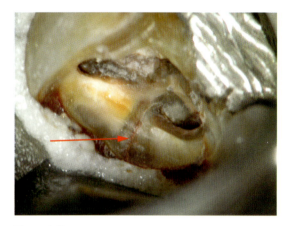

**Figure 1.40**

After cleaning the pulp floor and removing carious dentine, a crack was visible. The crack line extended from the mesial edge across the pulp floor and down into the orifice of a root canal. This tooth was unfortunately not saveable.

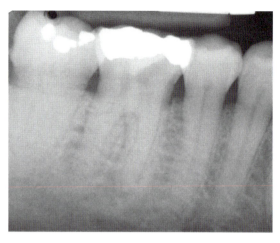

**Figure 1.41**

The mandibular first molar pulp has been extirpated, but the tooth still remains symptomatic. Careful analysis of the radiograph shows a periapical radiolucency that extends around both roots. This is often an indication of root fracture.

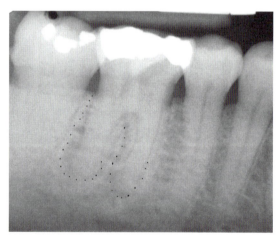

**Figure 1.42**

The periapical radiolucency highlighted with dots shows the area tracking around the lateral borders of the root.

disintegrating host cells have been implicated in failure.[48] Extrinsic factors may also be the cause of endodontic failure. Some root filling materials contain insoluble substances, e.g. talc-contaminated gutta percha cones. These can evoke foreign body reactions when protruding into the periradicular tissues and cause failure.[49] The cellulose component of paper points, cotton wool and some vegetables may also cause persistent inflammation.[50] This stable polysaccharide of plant cell walls is neither digested by man nor degraded by the defence cells. As a result, cellulose can remain in the tissues for long periods and elicit a foreign body reaction. Fragments of paper points can be dislodged or pushed beyond the apex. Leaving a tooth in open drainage is also

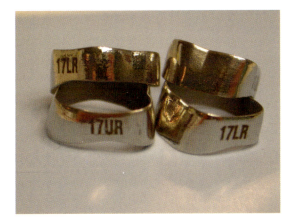

**Figure 1.43**

Plain orthodontic bands are an excellent means of stabilizing a fractured tooth and may prevent its demise during root canal treatment.

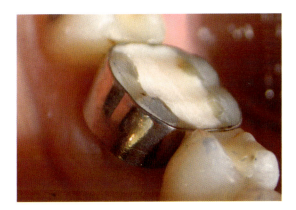

**Figure 1.44**

The band can be cemented to the tooth during treatment. If the tooth is severely broken down it will make rubber dam placement easier.

ill-advised as the root canal can become packed with food debris, small particles of which can eventually be forced into the periapical tissues.

Complications arising from such situations are often very difficult to treat. It is generally not possible to retrieve such material during non-surgical root canal retreatment and, therefore, if a tooth is symptomatic following an orthograde approach, surgery may be indicated.

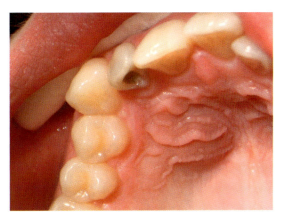

**Figure 1.45**

The maxillary right lateral incisor has an amalgam filling in the palatal surface and may well have been root treated. There is a large palatal swelling that appears to be located adjacent to the tooth. The central incisor and canine are not restored. It would appear quite likely that an infected root canal in the lateral incisor has resulted in the formation of an acute abscess. Before embarking on root canal retreatment it is essential to take a good periapical radiograph and carry out sensitivity testing of the adjacent teeth to confirm the diagnosis. Teeth can become non-vital as a result of trauma. Even though the coronal tooth substance may appear normal and the teeth do not have any restorations in place, the root canal can become infected at a later date via microcracks.

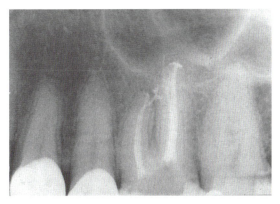

**Figure 1.46**

Complex root canal retreatment has been completed by an endodontist in the maxillary left first molar but the patient is in pain and is convinced that this tooth is the cause. Hot sensitivity testing reveals that the second molar is irreversibly pulpitic and requires root canal treatment.

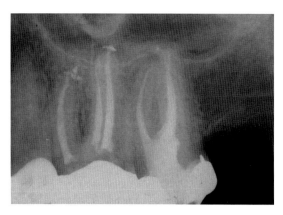

**Figure 1.47**

Following simple root canal treatment the patient is symptom-free. Root canal retreatment of the first molar would have been extremely difficult and would not have resolved the problem.

## HEALING WITH SCAR

Healing with scar or fibrous healing is not normally considered failure. It most commonly occurs following surgical endodontics, especially when the buccal and lingual plates have been perforated by an existing lesion. The result is an irregular resolution of the previous radiolucent area.

## NEUROPATHIC PROBLEMS

Neuropathic pain is defined by the International Association for the Study of Pain (IASP) as 'pain initiated or caused by a primary lesion or dysfunction in the nervous system'. Causal factors include injury, infection and surgery.

Commonly the term 'atypical facial pain' has been used to compartmentalize medically unexplained chronic facial pain. Phantom tooth pain (PTP) can occur following dental or surgical procedures such as root canal treatment, root end surgery or exodontias.[51] Other facial trauma or surgical procedures may have preceded the onset of PTP, the condition being characterized primarily by persistent pain. No amount of additional root canal treatment, root end surgery or exodontia will alleviate the problem.

Marbach et al reported continued pain for more than 1 month following root canal treatment in 7% of individuals. Of this sample, 3–6% showed signs of PTP. Tooth pain prior to root canal treatment appeared to be a risk factor for PTP.[52] The diagnostic criteria for PTP are as follows:

- the pain is in the face or described as toothache
- the pain is described as a constant deep, dull ache (some patients have a sharp pain that overlays the ache)
- a brief pain-free period is reported upon waking and there are no refractory periods
- pain develops (or continues) within 1 month of endodontic treatment, tooth extraction, trauma or medical procedure on the face
- there is an area of hyperalgesia overlying the area of treatment either on the face or intraorally
- sleep is undisturbed
- no radiographic or laboratory tests suggest other sources of pain.

A differential diagnosis would include trigeminal neuralgia, postherpetic neuralgia, acute herpes zoster and myofascial pain. Although there are no randomized controlled clinical trials for PTP, the anticonvulsant gabapentin has been successful for the treatment of phantom limb pain and is probably the drug of choice in the treatment of PTP.[53] Other drugs include tricyclic antidepressants, which may have an analgesic effect, nerve block anaesthesia and topical drugs such as capsaicin and clonidine.

The clinician should always be wary when there are no signs of endodontic pathology but a patient is convinced that a tooth requires root canal treatment, especially if multiple treatments have already been completed with no relief of symptoms.

## ECONOMIC CONSTRAINTS

Poor remuneration and the time constraints experienced by practitioners are often cited as the reason for poor-quality root canal treatment.[13] Providing high-quality endodontic treatment is time-consuming. Attempting to achieve the desired goals too fast results in basic biological treatment aims not being met. This in turn will undoubtedly result in endodontic failure. Interestingly, the method of remuneration does not appear to make a great difference to the quality of root canal treatment when measured in a global context.

## CONCLUSION

The main reasons for failure of primary root canal treatment are biological. Therefore, the rationale for retreatment has to be based on the sound biological objectives of elimination and future exclusion of infection from the root canal system.

The importance of careful and skilled technique when completing primary treatment of teeth with periapical periodontitis, and hence infected root canals, is highlighted. Iatrogenic problems causing inadequate cleaning of the root canal during primary treatment may lead to persistent infection and further difficulty if retreatment is required.

Adequate disinfection of the root canal system should allow the balance to tip in favour of periapical healing and success. To achieve this, existing materials, blockages and iatrogenic difficulties will have to be removed and overcome.

## REFERENCES

1. Sjögren U, Hagglund B, Sundqvist G, Wing K. Factors affecting the long-term results of endodontic treatment. *Journal of Endodontics* 1990; **16:** 498–504.
2. Dummer PM. The quality of root canal treatment in the general dental services. *Journal of the Dental Practice Board England and Wales* 1998; **19:** 8–10.
3. Saunders WP, Saunders EM, Sadiq J, Cruickshank E. Technical standard of root canal treatment in an adult Scottish sub-population. *British Dental Journal* 1997; **182:** 382–386.
4. Buckley M, Spangberg L. The prevalence and technical standard of endodontic treatment in an American sub-population. *Oral Surgery, Oral Medicine, Oral Pathology* 1995; **79:** 92–100.
5. De Cleen M, Schuurs A, Wesselink P, Wu MK. Periapical status and prevalence of endodontic treatment in an adult Dutch population. *International Endodontic Journal* 1993; **26:** 112–119.
6. Eckerbom M, Anderson JE, Magnasson T. Frequency and technical standard of endodontic treatment in a Swedish population. *Endodontics and Dental Traumatology* 1987; **3:** 245–248.
7. Lin LM, Pascon EA, Skribner J, Gaengler P, Langeland K. Clinical, radiographic, and treatment failures. *Oral Surgery, Oral Medicine, Oral Pathology, Oral Radiology and Endodontics* 1991; **71:** 603–611.
8. Siqueira JF Jr, Araújo MCP, Filho PFG, Fraga RC, Saboia Dantas CJ. Histological evaluation of the effectiveness of five instrumentation techniques for cleaning the apical third of root canals. *Journal of Endodontics* 1997; **23:** 499–502.
9. Kersten HW, Wesselink PR, Thoden Van Velzen SK. The diagnostic reliability of the buccal radiograph after root canal filling. *International Endodontic Journal* 1987; **20:** 20–24.
10. Sundqvist G, Figdor D, Persson S, Sjögren U. Microbiologic analysis of teeth with failed endodontic treatment and the outcome of conservative re-treatment. *Oral Surgery, Oral Medicine, Oral Pathology, Oral Radiology and Endodontics* 1998; **85:** 86–93.
11. Molander A, Reit C, Dahlén G, Kvist T. Microbiological status of root-filled teeth with apical periodontitis. *International Endodontic Journal* 1998; **31:** 1–7.
12. Marshall K, Page J. The use of rubber dam in the UK, a survey. *British Dental Journal* 1990; **169:** 286–291.
13. Stewardson DA. Endodontic standards in general dental practice – A survey in Birmingham, UK, Part 2. *European Journal of Prosthodontics and Restorative Dentistry* 2001; **9:** 113–116.
14. Bystrom A, Sundqvist G. The antibacterial action of sodium hypochlorite and EDTA in 60 cases of endodontic therapy.

*International Endodontic Journal* 1985; **18:** 35–40.

15. Mullaney TP. Instrumentation of finely curved canals. *Dental Clinics of North America* 1979; **23:** 575–585.

16. Goerig AC, Michelich RJ, Schultz HH. Instrumentation of root canals in molar teeth using the step-down technique. *Journal of Endodontics* 1982; **8:** 550–554.

17. Buchanan LS. The standardized-taper root canal preparation – Part 1 Concepts for variably tapered shaping instruments. *International Endodontic Journal* 2000; **33:** 516–529.

18. Al Shalabi RM, Omer OE, Glennon J. Root canal anatomy of maxillary first and second permanent molars. *International Endodontic Journal* 2000; **33:** 405–414.

19. Benjamin KA, Dowson J. Incidence of two root canals in human mandibular incisor teeth. *Oral Surgery, Oral Medicine, Oral Pathology, Oral Radiology and Endodontics* 1974; **38:** 122–126.

20. Pitt Ford TR, Rhodes JS, Pitt Ford HE. *Endodontics – problem solving in clinical practice.* London: Martin Dunitz; 2002.

21. Sequeira JF. Aetiology of root canal treatment failure: why well-treated teeth can fail. *International Endodontic Journal* 2001; **34:** 1–10.

22. Lee SJ, Monsef M, Torabinejad M. Sealing ability of a mineral trioxide aggregate for repair of lateral root perforations. *Journal of Endodontics* 1993; **19:** 541–544.

23. Firas Daoudi M. Microscopic management of endodontic procedural errors: perforation repair. *Dental Update* 2001; **28:** 176–180.

24. Strindberg LZ. The dependence of the results of pulp therapy on certain factors. *Acta Odontologica Scandinavica* 1956; **14:** 1–175.

25. Muruzábal M, Erasquin J, Devoto FCH. A study of periapical overfilling in root canal treatment in the molar of rat. *Archives of Oral Biology* 1966; **11:** 373–383.

26. Barbosa SV, Araki K, Spangberg LSW. Cytotoxicity of some modified root canal sealers and their leachable components. *Oral Surgery, Oral Medicine, Oral Pathology, Oral Radiology and Endodontics* 1993; **75:** 357–361.

27. Lin LM, Skribner JE, Gaengler P. Factors associated with endodontic treatment failures. *Journal of Endodontics* 1992; **18:** 625–627.

28. Sjögren U, Figdor D, Persson S, Sundqvist G. Influence of infection at the time of root filling on the outcome of endodontic treatment of teeth with apical periodontitis. *International Endodontic Journal* 1997; **30:** 297–306.

29. Yusuf H. The significance of the presence of foreign material periapically as a cause of failure of root treatment. *Oral Surgery, Oral Medicine, Oral Pathology, Oral Radiology and Endodontics* 1982; **54:** 566–574.

30. Saunders WP, Saunders EM. Coronal leakage as a cause of failure in root canal therapy: a review. *Endodontics and Dental Traumatology* 1994; **10:** 105–108.

31. Ray HA, Trope M. Periapical status of endodontically treated teeth in relation to the technical quality of the root filling and the coronal restoration. *International Endodontic Journal* 1995; **28:** 12–18.

32. Kirkevang LL, Ørstavik D, Hörsted-Bindslev P, Wenzel A. Periapical status and quality of root fillings in a Danish population. *International Endodontic Journal* 2000; **33:** 509–511.

33. Ricucci D, Bergenholtz G. Bacterial status in root-filled teeth exposed to the oral environment by loss of restoration and fracture or caries – a histobacteriological study of treated cases. *International Endodontic Journal* 2003; **36:** 787–802.

34. Siren EK, Haapsalo MPP, Ranta K. Microbiological findings and clinical treatment procedures in endodontic cases selected for microbiological investigation. *International Endodontic Journal* 1997; **30:** 91–95.

35. Molander A, Reit C, Dahlen G. Microbiological status of root-filled teeth with apical periodontitis. *International Endodontic Journal* 1998; **31:** 1–7.

36. Sundqvist G, Figdor D, Persson S. Microbiologic analysis of teeth with failed endodontic treatment and the outcome of conservative re-treatment. *Oral Surgery, Oral Medicine, Oral Pathology, Oral Radiology and Endodontics* 1998; **85:** 86–93.

37. Hommez GMG, Verhelst R, Claeys G, Vaneechotte M, De Moor RJG. Investigation of the effect of the coronal restoration on the composition of the root canal microflora in teeth with apical periodontitis by means of T-RFLP analysis. *International Endodontic Journal* 2004; **37:** 819–827.

38. Nair PNR, Sjogren U, Kahnberg KE. Intraradicular bacteria and fungi in root-filled, asymptomatic human teeth with therapy-resistant periapical lesions: a long-term light and electron microscopic follow-up study. *Journal of Endodontics* 1990; **16:** 580–588.

39. Waltimo TMT, Orstavik D, Sirén EK, Haapasalo MPP. In vitro susceptibility of *Candida albicans* to four disinfectants and their combinations. *International Endodontic Journal* 1999; **32:** 42–49.

40. Sundqvist G, Reuterving CO. Isolation of *Actinomyces israelii* from periapical lesion. *Journal of Endodontics* 1980; **6:** 602–606.

41. Nair PNR. Periapical actinomycosis. *Journal of Endodontics* 1984; **12:** 567–570.

42. Sjögren U, Happonen RP, Kahnberg KE, Sundqvist G. Survival of *Arachnia propionica* in periapical tissue. *International Endodontic Journal* 1988; **21:** 277–282.

43. Sakellariou PL. Periapical actinomycosis: report of a case and review of the literature. *Endodontics and Dental Traumatology* 1996; **12:** 151–154.

44. Costerton JW, Lewandowski Z, Debeer D, Caldwell D, Korber D, James G. Biofilms: the customized microniche. *Journal of Bacteriology* 1994; **176:** 2137–2147.

45. Tronstad L, Barnett F, Cervone F. Periapical bacterial plaque in teeth refractory to endodontic treatment. *Endodontics and Dental Traumatology* 1990; **6:** 73–77.

46. Siqueira Jf Jr, Lopes HP. Bacteria on the apical root surfaces of untreated teeth with periradicular lesions: a scanning electron microscopy study. *International Endodontic Journal* 2001 **34:** 617–627.

47. Nair PNR, Sjögren U, Figdor D, Sundqvist G. Persistent periapical radiolucencies of root-filled human teeth, failed endodontic treatments, and periapical scars. *Oral Surgery, Oral Medicine, Oral Pathology, Oral Radiology and Endodontics* 1999; **87:** 617–627.

48. Nair PNR, Sjögren U, Sundqvist G. Cholesterol crystals as an etiological factor in non-resolving chronic inflammation: an experimental study in guinea pigs. *European Journal of Oral Science* 1998; **106:** 644–650.

49. Nair PNR, Sjögren U, Krey G, Sundqvist G. Therapy-resistant foreign body giant cell granuloma at the periapex of a root-filled human tooth. *Journal of Endodontics* 1990; **16:** 589–595.

50. Simon JHS, Chimenti RA, Mintz CA. Clinical significance of the pulse granuloma. *Journal of Endodontics* 1982; **6:** 116–119.

51. Marbach JJ, Raphael KG. Phantom tooth pain: a new look at an old dilemma. *Pain Medicine* 2000; **1:** 68–77.

52. Marbach JJ, Hulbrock J, Hohn C, Segal AG. Incidence of phantom tooth pain: an atypical facial neuralgia. *Oral Surgery, Oral Medicine, Oral Pathology* 1982; **53:** 190–193.

53. Rowbotham M, Harden N, Stacey B, Bernstein P, Magnus-Miller L. Gabapentin for the treatment of postherpetic neuralgia: a randomized controlled trial. *JAMA* 1998; **280:** 1837–1842.

# 2 DECISION MAKING AND TREATMENT PLANNING

CONTENTS • Introduction • What is success? • Clinical Guidelines of the European Society of Endodontics • Decision Making • Decision Making and Treatment Planning Process • Decision-making Factors Affecting Outcome • Treatment Planning • Conclusion • References

## INTRODUCTION

Although outcomes of endodontic treatment have been of interest for many years, there is an apparent disparity between the success rates reported by cross-sectional studies (31–60%) and those of longitudinal studies (85–95%). Much of the published data have been gleaned from retrospective, non-randomized cohorts. Ideally such studies would be conducted prospectively and the factor of interest randomized. For ethical and practical reasons, this is generally not possible. There are several possible explanations for the discrepancy in outcomes, such as variation between studies in terms of sample size, definition of success, treatment procedures, recall rate, length of observation period and radiographic interpretation. In this respect, the conclusions drawn from original historical data may be biased. More recently, meta-analysis and systematic reviews have been used to assimilate the data provided by multiple studies and will hopefully improve the body of evidence available for clinical use.

## WHAT IS SUCCESS?

### Patient Viewpoint

A patient may consider success as relief from acute symptoms, perhaps the resolution of swelling or absence of tenderness. Patients will probably be unaware of a chronic lesion that may, with little warning (and usually at the most inconvenient time), transform from a dormant state into an acute problem (Figures 2.1–2.3).

### The Clinical Viewpoint

Traditionally, success has been determined by lack of any symptoms and a normal radiological presentation, while any visible or radiological signs of disease indicate failure. It was the research published by Strindberg in 1956[1] that incorporated a system of criteria for assessment of success and failure based on the presence or absence of periapical rarefaction

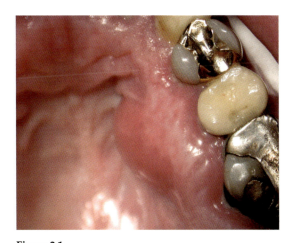

**Figure 2.1**

The patient may consider success as relief from acute symptoms such as gross swelling.

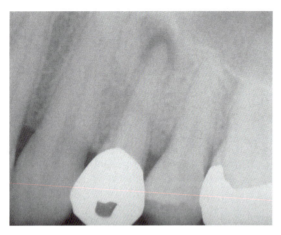

**Figure 2.2**

In this case the maxillary left first premolar has chronic periapical periodontitis associated with it. An attempt at root canal treatment has been made but the root canals are extremely fine and have not been successfully negotiated. It is likely that following access cavity preparation coronal leakage has resulted in complete microbial colonization of the root canal system. The patient is symptom-free. The patient is made aware of the risk of acute exacerbation should the tooth not be treated. The prognosis for a non-surgical approach should be good. Root-end surgery would not be appropriate due to the infected root canals.

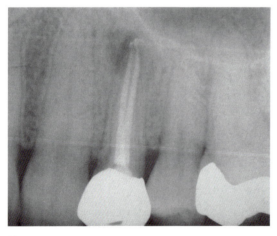

**Figure 2.3**

The completed root canal retreatment. Sclerosed root canals can normally be located under high magnification with a microscope and, once located, careful preparation will enable them to be enlarged, irrigated and then sealed.

**Table 2.1** *Strindberg criteria for success and failure*

| | Radiographic findings |
|---|---|
| Success | The contours' width and structure of the periodontal margin were normal<br>The periodontal contours were widened mainly around an existing filling |
| Uncertain | Technically unsatisfactory or ambiguous control radiographs that for some reason could not be repeated<br>The tooth was extracted prior to 3-year follow-up |
| Failure | A decrease in the size of periapical rarefaction<br>An unchanged periradicular rarefaction<br>An appearance of a new rarefaction or increase in previous rarefaction |

(Table 2.1). Strindberg considered that the presence of periapical radiolucency after a period of 4 years following root canal treatment would indicate signs of biological failure. It is interesting to note however, that complete healing sometimes took up to 10 years.

Clinical evaluation of the patient will determine whether there are any signs of disease, such as swelling, sinus tracts, tenderness on biting and mobility. The presenting symptoms are also gauged, but as a subjective assessment; the absence of symptoms does not necessarily mean absence of disease. Since clinical symptoms tend to occur infrequently, biological evaluation nearly always has to rely on radiographic findings.

## Histological Viewpoint

Histological assessment of an endodontically treated tooth may offer the ultimate standard for determining success or failure. But it would obviously not be feasible or ethical in the clinical environment to take surgical block sections of all root-treated teeth for microscopic analysis.

The question for any clinician is whether a situation that may appear healthy (and symptom-free) on a macroscopic scale could show signs of inflammation and failure at a cellular or microscopic level.

## CLINICAL GUIDELINES OF THE EUROPEAN SOCIETY OF ENDODONTICS

The European Society of Endodontics Guidelines indicate that root-filled teeth should be reviewed radiographically at 1 year and then subsequently as required for up to 4 years to assess whether treatment has been successful.[2] Success would be indicated by relief from symptoms, healing of sinus tracts and reduction or complete resolution of periapical radiolucency. If a root-filled tooth is functional, clinically symptomless and has no evidence of disease radiographically, then treatment can be considered a success (Table 2.2).

Reit and co-workers systematically studied the decision-making process with regard to retreatment. They suggest that patients should be assessed for outcome of treatment 1 year postoperatively and, if in doubt, recalled 3 years later.[3]

## DECISION MAKING

The decision-making process for endodontic retreatment can be complex. This is perhaps highlighted by the substantial variation that has been recorded amongst clinicians in the management of endodontically treated teeth with symptom-free periapical lesions.[4,5] Unfortunately, much of the decision-making process appears to lend itself to rather heuristic principles, as subjective influences affect treatment planning decisions. Various aspects of the endodontic retreatment decision-making process have been explored.[6,7] Factors contributing to differences in decision-making processes amongst groups of clinicians include the dentist, the patient, cost, environmental resources, clinical experience, training and speciality.

It has been hypothesized that clinicians view the disease process as a health scale continuum and that variation in instigating intervention can be considered to result from individuals having differing cut-off points along the scale. This was developed as the 'praxis concept theory', which proposed that dentists perceive periapical lesions of varying sizes as different stages on a continuous health scale based on their radiographic appearance.[8]

Table 2.2 *Diagnosis of success and failure*

|  | Clinical | Radiological |
|---|---|---|
| Success | There is no tenderness to palpation or percussion<br>Normal mobility and function<br>No sinus tract or periodontal defect<br>No signs of inflammation<br>No pain or discomfort | Contours, width and structure of periodontal ligament space are normal<br>The periodontal ligament contours are widened around excess filling material |
| Mixed | Sporadic or vague symptoms that are most often not reproducible<br>Feeling of pressure or tightness<br>Slight discomfort when chewing or pressing on tooth with finger or tongue | The periapical area has not changed in size<br>The periodontal ligament space does not look completely normal |
| Failure | Persistent symptoms<br>Recurrent sinus tract swelling or pain<br>Pain on percussion or palpation<br>Mobility or function that is not normal | The periapical area has not changed in size or has enlarged<br>The appearance of new periapical or lateral radiolucency<br>Maximum review time 4 years |

It has also been suggested that variation in treatment decisions stems essentially from two main sources, perceptual variation and judgemental variation.[9] Perceptual variation may affect the actual process of diagnosis. Judgemental variation relates to the application of treatment once it has been established that disease is present. The judgement of dentists is affected by various factors such as their own individual treatment threshold and their attitudes to risk, as well as patient and environmental factors. It has been postulated that guidelines could be compiled for planning root canal retreatment in an attempt to reduce operator variation. Some authors however, consider that variation is not necessarily undesirable[10] and that failure to adhere to strict guidelines may increase the risk of litigation. In addition, there is a danger that didactic guidelines could stifle innovation and enterprise, which are vital to the continuing development of the knowledge base.

Ultimately the decision whether to retreat or not is made between a clinician and the patient following presentation of all the factors on both sides. Theoretical and practical knowledge of the clinican as well as the perosnal and moral values of both parties are all taken into account. Every situation will be unique and therefore the eventual outcome will reflect this. Variation in prescription within normal boundaries and ethical practice should perhaps not be perceived as a problem.

If root canal treatment has failed, there are usually five possible treatment options:

• review or do nothing
• root canal retreatment
• root end surgery
• extraction
• referral.

### Review or do Nothing

There may be occasions where a conservative approach is appropriate. The balance of factors to consider in a case of failed root canal treatment, where review is considered, include an assessment of the risk of future disease against the risk of leaving untreated disease. One of the most difficult decisions is whether to retreat a root-filled tooth that requires a crown when it shows no evidence of a defective core or periapical disease and is symptom-free but has a technically deficient root canal filling (e.g. inappropriate filling material or the root filling is short). It is sometimes very difficult to judge how much improvement can be gained by retreatment when difficulties are expected in carrying out the treatment (e.g. negotiating a ledge).

The natural history of periapical lesions in root-filled teeth is not well known and information from many studies is inconclusive.[1,11–13] It is difficult to predict the impact of retreatment in the population as a whole but root canal infection as a systemic health hazard is considered to be a low risk for the medically uncompromised individual. As a consequence, refraining from active treatment can be a legitimate treatment modality.[14,15] The majority of treated cases that develop apical periodontitis will do so within 1 year.[16] Failure after 1 year is infrequent and therefore observation at this time will, in the majority of cases, give a good indication of outcome (Figures 2.4–2.7).

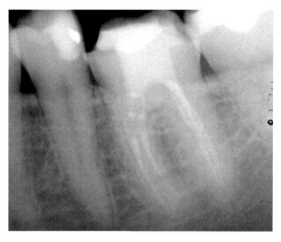

**Figure 2.4**

The mandibular left first molar has recently been root filled. Four root canals were located, shaped, cleaned and obturated. The root filling is of good quality and there are no radiographic signs of periapical pathology. The patient is still experiencing mild symptoms of discomfort on biting. In this case reviewing the situation would be appropriate as the previous treatment has only just been completed. Transient inflammation following initial root canal treatment could be causing the patient's symptoms. It is probably worth checking that the tooth is not in hyper-occlusion (which is unlikely in this case).

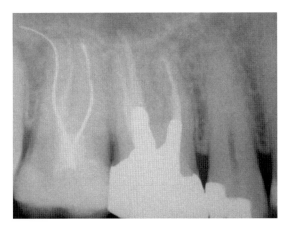

**Figure 2.5**

Although root canal retreatment was carried out on the maxillary right first molar, the maxillary right second molar was placed under review. The root filling is grossly over-extended in the distobuccal canal and a dated silver point technique has been used to obturate the canals. There is little radiological evidence of periapical pathology. The tooth is symptom-free and the coronal restoration is reasonable. A new restoration is not intended as part of the overall treatment plan and it would therefore be quite appropriate to place the tooth under review. Root canal retreatment of such a root filling would be challenging.

Review may be considered when:

- the tooth is symptom-free
- there is no systemic risk by no intervention
- there are no signs of inflammation or infection
- the tooth does not require a new restoration
- root canal treatment has only recently been completed and the outcome is uncertain.

## Root Canal Retreatment

Root canal retreatment is often the preferred means of treating a failed root canal procedure, especially when the failure is due to a technical deficiency.

The existing root filling is removed and the infected root canal disinfected using irrigants and medicaments. Root canal retreatment is often much more complicated than initial treatment as restorations may need to be dismantled in order to gain access to the canal system. It is important to assess whether the tooth is restorable prior to embarking on

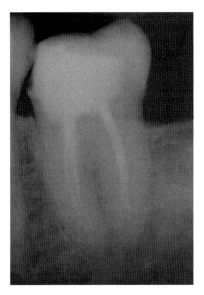

**Figure 2.6**

Root canal treatment of this mandibular left first molar was completed approximately 6 months previously. The root filling is slightly short in all root canals. However, a fair attempt has been made to shape the canals and hopefully disinfect them. A periapical area on the distal root has decreased slightly in size and the tooth is symptom-free. In this situation, it would be reasonable to review the tooth for a further 6 months. If healing does not appear to be occurring at 1 year, then root canal retreatment would probably be undertaken. A cusp coverage restoration should be provided when healing is evident.

prolonged and often expensive treatment. If a tooth is unrestorable, then it should be extracted and a suitable replacement provided (Figure 2.8).

The risks encountered during retreatment must be considered. These include possible weakening of the existing tooth substance, damage to existing coronal restoration, difficulties in removing posts or existing root fillings and the challenge of negotiating iatrogenic difficulties. These risks are presented to the patient, included in the decision-making process and accepted by both parties before embarking on treatment. An element of personal preference may also have an effect on the decision-making process because of factors such as knowledge, experience and even dental school policy (Figure 2.9).

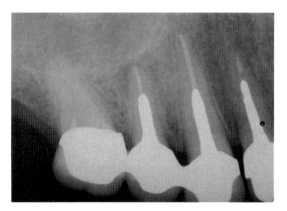

**Figure 2.7**

The teeth in the maxillary right quadrant have been restored using splinted crowns. The canine and pre-molar teeth have been root filled and post cores cemented. The patient is symptom-free and there are no abnormal clinical signs. Radiographically, the root fillings look good but there is a periapical radiolucency associated with the second premolar. Non-surgical retreatment would be highly complex and risk irreversible damage to the new bridgework. A surgical approach may be appropriate if healing does not occur. As root canal treatment was only recently completed, this case will be reviewed.

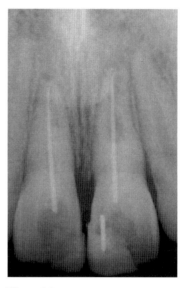

**Figure 2.9**

Root canal retreatment of these maxillary central incisors in a young adult should be relatively simple as the single cone root filings can be easily removed. It is important to try and retain such teeth if an alternative such as an implant solution is to be considered in the long term.

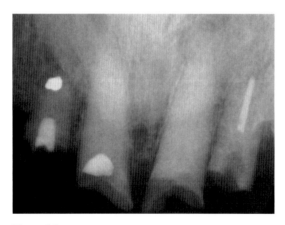

**Figure 2.8**

The lateral incisor teeth have been root filled and in the maxillary right lateral incisor an amalgam root end filling has been placed. Post crown restorations would have a guarded prognosis as the root length is short, and the patient is completely edentulous in the posterior segments. It would be appropriate in this case to consider alternative treatment options such as an overdenture or perhaps an implant-supported prosthesis.

Root canal retreatment is normally indicated when:

- conventional root canal treatment has failed
- there are signs of inflammation or infection associated with a root-filled tooth
- there are persistent symptoms from a root-filled tooth, or the presence of a sinus tract, swelling or pain
- a root-filled tooth has failed for technical reasons
- there is systemic risk if no intervention is made
- the tooth is restorable
- the tooth has evidence of periapical radio-lucency and requires a new restoration
- the existing root filling is technically deficient and a new restoration is required
- the patient conserts to retreatment.

## Root End Surgery

A surgical approach is normally reserved for cases in which apparently good-quality root

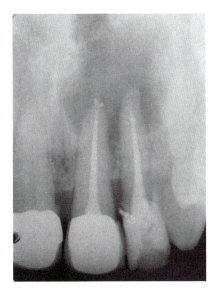

**Figure 2.10**

In some situations root end surgery may be considered in combination with root canal retreatment. In this case a large radicular cyst was present above the maxillary left central and lateral incisors. Root canal retreatment was completed prior to surgery.

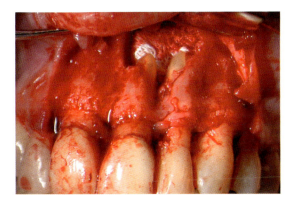

**Figure 2.11**

The radicular cyst was removed surgically.

canal treatment or retreatment has been unsuccessful. This is because the placement of a root-end filling in a tooth with an infected root canal will undoubtedly lead to failure. A modern surgical approach is technically demanding (Figures 2.10, 2.11).

Root end surgery may be considered when:

- it is impractical to carry out conventional root canal retreatment, e.g. if a very large post

were well cemented in an already weakened root, resulting in a high risk of fracture on removal
- root canal treatment or non-surgical retreatment has been unsuccessful
- as an adjunct to root canal retreatment, perhaps in perforation repair or to remove extruded material
- when root or tooth resection is required
- when a biopsy is required
- for investigation and exploration, e.g. in a case of root fracture
- patient preference, following assessment of risk.

## Extraction

If a tooth is unrestorable or the prognosis for root canal retreatment is poor, extraction is the only option. As the prognosis for modern root canal retreatment has become clearer, fewer teeth have been placed in this category (Figure 2.12).

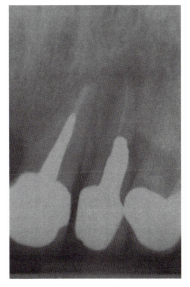

**Figure 2.12**

The post that has been cemented in this lateral incisor perforates the root wall. The root canal and perforation site are infected and there is direct communication with the oral cavity via a periodontal pocket. A better long-term prognosis may be offered by extracting the tooth and replacing it with a bridge or implant-supported restoration.

Extraction may be the treatment of choice:

- when the tooth or root is fractured and is not saveable
- if an alternative, such as removable or fixed bridgework or an implant-based solution, would offer a better prognosis
- when the patient elects not to have retreatment when all options have been explained
- when root canal retreatment is unlikely to be successful.

### Referral

There are specialist practitioners who have additional expertise in the retreatment of endodontic failures. Surgical and non-surgical procedures are often technically demanding and the results achieved dependent on operator skill. Complicated cases may be preferentially referred to a specialist or highly experienced colleague.

Referral may be appropriate when:

- the clinician is unable to make a diagnosis
- access is limited
- root canal treatment has failed
- retreatment has failed
- complexity of treatment is greater than the clinician's expertise
- surgical endodontic treatment is required
- patients present with complex medical histories
- combined multidisciplinary problems
- patient requests referral.

## DECISION MAKING AND TREATMENT PLANNING PROCESS

There are several phases that are involved in eventually arriving at a final treatment plan. First, the clinician should complete a thorough, methodical history and examination of the patient, which includes any necessary radiographs and special tests. From the pooled information, a preliminary diagnosis can be made. The root filling will be confirmed as a success, failure or uncertain diagnosis. The clinician now balances the multitude of variables that contribute to the assessment of risk. The outcome will be one of the following options:

- further investigation problem not endodontic in origin

- review
- non-surgical retreatment
- root end surgery
- referral
- extraction.

Treatment planning can then be undertaken. (History, examination and special tests are covered in detail in Chapter 1 of *Endodontics: problem solving in clinical practice*, TR Pitt Ford, JS Rhodes, HE Pitt Ford (eds). London: Martin Dunitz; 2003.)

### Clinical Assessment

With respect to root canal retreatment, several factors regarding previous treatment are of interest.

### What Treatment Has Been Provided?

Sometimes root canal treatment may have already been attempted several times. The root canals of teeth that have been left open to drain for a considerable length of time are often packed with food debris and may also become saturated with bacterial colonies. These cases will be difficult to disinfect. Information divulged by the patient may highlight likely problems that could be incurred during retreatment. However, patients can become confused or uncertain about specific details when extensive treatment has been carried out, and it is not uncommon in this situation to find that the patient has forgotten that a particular tooth has even been root filled.

### Why Was It Carried Out?

Was the patient in pain? Have the original presenting symptoms been improved or changed as a result of the treatment?

### When Was It Completed?

If the root filling has only recently been completed, then it may be too early to ascertain whether it is failing. The timing of original treatment may give an indication of the techniques and materials that have been used. The operator must remember that a single radiograph gives a 'snap shot' in time and does not provide any historical information.

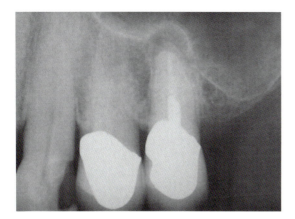

**Figure 2.13**

Root canal retreatment of the maxillary left second premolar was completed by an endodontist. The tooth was subsequently restored using a post core and crown. There is a small periapical area present and the tooth is occasionally symptomatic. The root filling and restoration are excellent and therefore a surgical approach was considered more appropriate in this case.

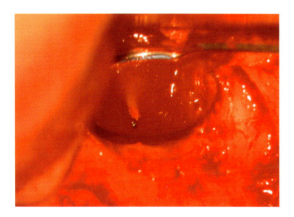

**Figure 2.14**

A view of the resected root end during surgery showing the well-condensed gutta percha root filling, and a small piece of separated instrument not visible on the radiograph.

## Who Carried Out the Previous Treatment?

If an experienced practitioner or specialist has had difficulty gaining access to canals or instrumenting to length, will further attempts improve things? Would it be more appropriate to consider a surgical approach? (Figures 2.13–2.15).

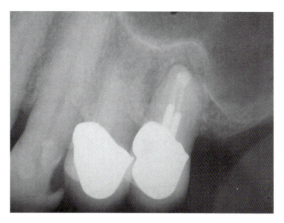

**Figure 2.15**

The completed root end surgery. The patient is now symptom-free.

## Where Was It Carried Out?

The methodology and philosophy of treatment vary considerably between different nations. It is not uncommon to find patients who have travelled the globe and have received treatment in many different countries. Some root filling pastes used in former Eastern Block countries are notoriously difficult to remove.

### Special Tests

Even though the clinician may suspect a particular root-filled tooth to have failed, it is good practice to confirm the diagnosis with special tests. Sensitivity testing of adjacent teeth and occasionally teeth from the opposing arch may be required to clearly identify the culprit. Combining the results of special tests and radiographic reports will help compound the evidence. Primary root canal treatment is generally much easier to complete than retreatment, and misdiagnosis could be expensive (Figures 2.16–2.18).

### Radiological Examination

Standardized radiographs taken using a paralleling device and developed to a high quality are used to assess the quality of the previous root filling. In particular they can be used to

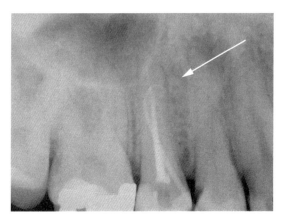

**Figure 2.16**

In this case a patient presented complaining of toothache in the maxillary right quadrant that appeared to be originating from the maxillary second premolar. A gutta percha point placed in a buccal sinus tract appeared to be pointing to the root-filled tooth. Sensitivity testing of the adjacent teeth revealed that the maxillary right first premolar was in fact non-vital and there was evidence of periapical radiolucency around the root tips.

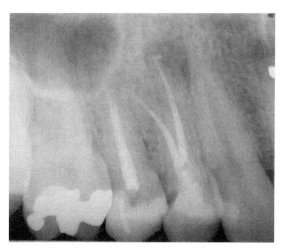

**Figure 2.18**

The case has been completed and, following shaping and cleaning, the sinus tract completely healed. Failure to carry out sensitivity testing would not have revealed the true cause of the patient's symptoms and retreatment of the maxillary right second premolar would not have resolved matters.

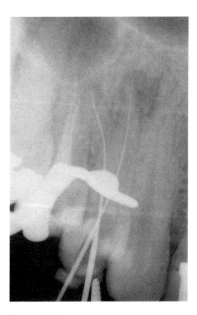

**Figure 2.17**

A diagnostic root length estimation radiograph reveals that the palatal root of the maxillary right first premolar extends over the apex of the maxillary right second premolar.

check for the correct material and length, and if the material is well condensed. The periodontal ligament space can be traced around the root. An increase in width, either laterally or apically, may indicate the presence of a localized inflammatory response. There may be a defined radiolucency in close association with the root. The location, size and nature of any radiolucencies are recorded.

It is sometimes helpful to take radiographs from different angles to ascertain whether canals have been missed. It is also possible to identify which root canal contains a fractured instrument (Figures 2.19–2.21).

A methodical and meticulous approach to the assessment of radiographs allows the practitioner to detect any conditions that are not consistent with normal, healthy anatomy. In addition, the clinician should always be careful to try to avoid subjective variation. Strict scoring systems such as the periapical index (PAI),[17] which enable some degree of standardization in scientific research, could perhaps be adapted for use in clinical practice in ensuring quality control and for clinical audit (Figure 2.22).

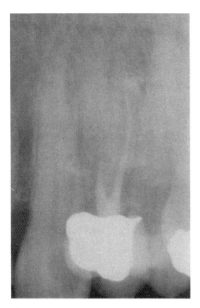

**Figure 2.19**

Taking a radiograph from an angle can help indicate whether there are missed root canals. In this case the radiograph has been taken from a mesial aspect to show both root canals in a maxillary premolar. The buccal canal has been obturated to the full extent. However, the palatal canal is under-prepared and under-filled.

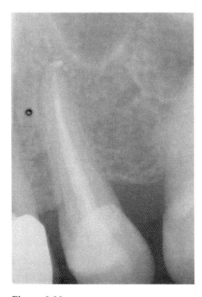

**Figure 2.20**

A periapical radiograph of a root-filled maxillary first premolar shows excellent root filling.

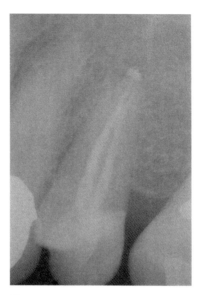

**Figure 2.21**

By taking an angled view, the root canals can be separated and visualized individually. The filling material is short in one canal and there is a fractured instrument tip present.

Previous radiographs are valuable for providing comparisons and historical information. If a lesion has not decreased in size, root canal treatment may not necessarily be considered to have failed. Further review could be required, and this process may continue for up to 4 years.

## DECISION-MAKING FACTORS AFFECTING OUTCOME

### Periapical Periodontitis

The only factor that has consistently been proven to influence the outcome of endodontic treatment is the presence of apical periodontitis. It has been shown that the success rate for root canal retreatment is approximately 15–20% higher in teeth without periapical lesions than in those with apical periodontitis (Table 2.3).

Following a sound biological approach to root canal treatment, a success rate of 96% was achieved for root canal treatment in teeth with no lesion, whereas the presence of apical periodontitis resulted in a reduced success rate of 86%.[21] In the same study, the success rate for

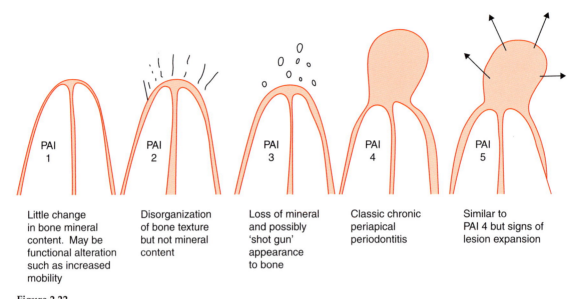

| PAI 1 | PAI 2 | PAI 3 | PAI 4 | PAI 5 |
|---|---|---|---|---|
| Little change in bone mineral content. May be functional alteration such as increased mobility | Disorganization of bone texture but not mineral content | Loss of mineral and possibly 'shot gun' appearance to bone | Classic chronic periapical periodontitis | Similar to PAI 4 but signs of lesion expansion |

**Figure 2.22**

Periapical index (PAI). Adapted with permission from Ørstavik et al.[17]

**Table 2.3** *Treatment success following endodontic retreatment in teeth with and without apical periodontitis*

| Author | Date | Apical periodontitis | Cases observed | Treatment success (%) |
|---|---|---|---|---|
| Molven and Halse[18] | 1988 | None | 76 | 89 |
| Molven and Halse[18] | 1989 | Present | 98 | 71 |
| Sjögren et al[19] | 1990 | None | 173 | 98 |
| Sjögren et al[19] | 1990 | Present | 94 | 62 |
| Friedman et al[20] | 1995 | None | 42 | 100 |
| Friedman et al[20] | 1995 | Present | 86 | 56 (uncertain 34; failed 10) |

root canal retreatment was shown to be 62%. In another study the presence of preoperative periapical radiolucency was shown to have a significant negative effect on the outcome of root canal retreatment, although overall success rates were high (91%).[22]

One can assume that the presence of a periapical area normally indicates bacterial infection of the root canal system. Retreatment cases often present with apical periodontitis and may be more difficult to disinfect effectively both from a technical point of view and as a result of the types of bacteria present. There is no room for missed canals, iatrogenic errors or complacency if a high success rate is

to be achieved when treating teeth with apical periodontitis.

## Length of Instrumentation and Obturating Material

Healing was reported in 94% of root-filled teeth where preparation and root filling ended within 0–2 mm of the radiographic apex.[19] Preparations that were shorter showed only 68% success. Another study showed that 55% of over-filled roots with defective seals were associated with apical periodontitis, whereas only 12% of root

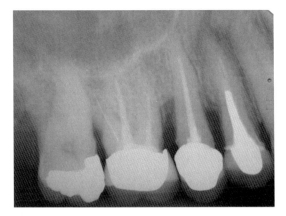

**Figure 2.23**

In this case the maxillary right premolar teeth have been root filled. The root-filling material is short of the root apex in both teeth. There is a periapical radiolucency associated with the maxillary first premolar. However, there is little evidence of periapical pathology associated with the maxillary second premolar.

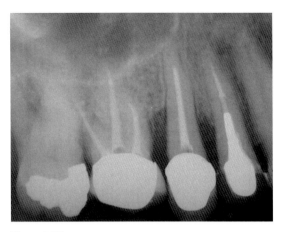

**Figure 2.25**

The completed case shows the canals obturated with gutta percha. As expected, root-filling material is short in the second premolar but the canals in the first premolar have been obturated to their full extent.

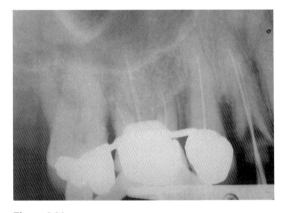

**Figure 2.24**

During root canal retreatment it was possible to regain patency in the root canals of the first premolar. This is important as the root canals are undoubtedly infected and should be disinfected to their full extent if possible. The second premolar was blocked apically and it was not possible to gain patency. This should not be of serious concern, as the tooth is not associated with periapical pathology and optimistically there will be little chance of residual bacteria in the apical portion.

fillings that ended within 0–2 mm of the radiographic apex showed periapical radiolucency.[23] The crux of the problem may be whether or not an infected canal was present before primary treatment (Figures 2.23–2.25).

As discussed previously, gutta percha is generally well tolerated by the tissues and does not initiate an inflammatory response per se. However, over-filling often occurs following over-preparation which, in the presence of an infected canal, may result in extrusion of infected debris and obturating material into the tissues. Likewise, under-filling, which may result from failing to instrument the canal completely, could result in bacteria remaining in the root canal following treatment. Both situations could subsequently lead to induction or persistence of periapical inflammation. In a recent study of teeth or roots with signs of apical periodontitis, a millimeter loss in working length increased the chance of treatment failure by 14%.[24]

The importance of thoroughly disinfecting the entire root canal system cannot be underestimated in teeth with periapical periodontitis and infected root canals. Ledged or blocked canals may prevent renegotiation of the canal and therefore adequate disinfection. A 2-year follow-up study showed a success rate of 86.8% for retreatment of teeth in which there were morphological changes as opposed to 47% in canals that had been altered by the previous treatment.[25] Obstruction that prevents complete negotiation may not always affect outcome.[26]

## Size of Periapical Radiolucency

The host osteolytic response has not been directly correlated with the extent of canal contamination by bacteria but it has been suggested that an increase in the size of periapical radiolucency beyond 5 mm diameter may have a negative effect on the outcome of root canal treatment.[22,27] The converse has also been reported. This may be due to the fact that root canal-treated teeth associated with large areas take longer to heal and require further observation.

## Technical Factors

Failure of root canal treatment following procedural inadequacies is often an indication for root canal retreatment. However, technical factors can influence the difficulty of completing root canal retreatment (Figures 2.26, 2.27).

## Fractured Instruments and Silver Points

Instruments that have fractured coronally are easier to remove than those positioned more apically. If the instrument is visible with good

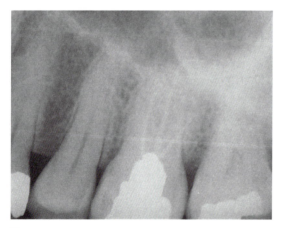

**Figure 2.26**

A maxillary first molar has been root filled using a single cone technique but remains symptomatic. The canals are under-prepared and the filling material is short in all of them. As there is a technical deficiency in the primary treatment, root canal retreatment should have a good prognosis.

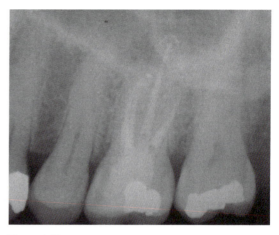

**Figure 2.27**

A missed second mesiobuccal canal was located during root canal retreatment. All the other canals were successfully renegotiated, shaped, cleaned and obturated. The patient is now symptom-free.

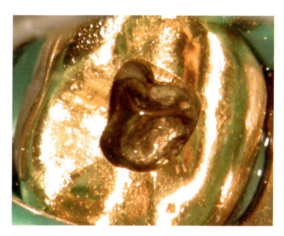

**Figure 2.28**

Leaving a tag of silver point in the core material should make removal considerably easier.

illumination and magnification, then removal is probably more likely. Nickel–titanium instruments tend to be more difficult to remove than stainless steel files (Figures 2.28–2.32).

## Types of Filling Material

Pastes usually offer the least resistance to removal, but some cements, such as phenol

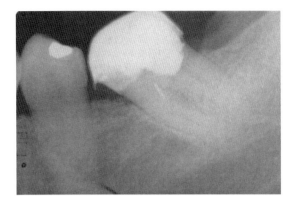

**Figure 2.29**

Removing a fractured instrument from the orifice of a root canal should be relatively simple. In this mandibular left molar, a fractured orifice opener can be seen in one of the mesiobuccal canals. It should be relatively simple to remove using ultrasonics. The tilting of the tooth made access more difficult.

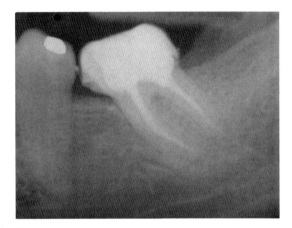

**Figure 2.30**

The previous case root canal retreated. The fragment of instrument was removed uneventfully and the root canals retreated.

resins, are extremely difficult to remove. Silver points are easier to remove when an extension has been left in the access cavity but can be much more difficult when there is restricted access or the head of the point is buried subgingivally. Single cone gutta percha fillings are generally easier to remove than well-compacted thermoplasticized fillings. Plastic Thermafil carriers can be removed relatively easily but those with a metal carrier can be more difficult.

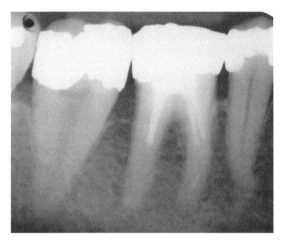

**Figure 2.31**

A fragment of file is retained in the apical part of a mesial canal of this mandibular right molar. The mesial canals have also been ledged. Root canal retreatment will be extremely difficult. It may not be possible to remove the fractured instrument. As there is a periapical area associated with this root, it is important to try to disinfect the canal as thoroughly as possible. There could potentially be an indication for endodontic surgery in this instance or an alternative such as fixed bridgework or an implant-based solution.

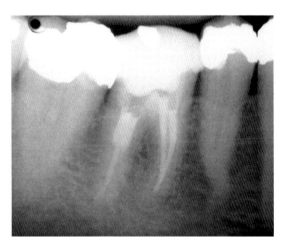

**Figure 2.32**

Fortunately, root canal retreatment was successful using a non-surgical approach. The ledges in the mesial canals were negotiated and the fragment of instrument removed. In the distal canal what initially appeared to be two separate canals was in fact one larger canal, and this has been completely prepared to the full length of the root.

## Perforations

Successful treatment of perforations depends on the operator's ability to seal the defect and prevent infection. The size, position and time of perforation all affect successful treatment. The earlier a perforation can be repaired, the better, and the possibility of infection must be kept to a minimum. Large perforations are most difficult to seal (>0.5 mm) and are associated with more tissue destruction. Perforations in close proximity to the gingival sulcus can lead to contamination by bacteria from the oral cavity. Perforations located below crestal bone have a better prognosis, as do those in the floor of the molar pulp chamber away from canal orifices. The introduction of Mineral Trioxide Aggregate has improved the outcome of perforation repair (Figures 2.33–2.36).[28]

## Restoration

The general state of restorations in the mouth may affect the decision as to whether root canal retreatment is advisable. Patients presenting with gross caries will require a preventative

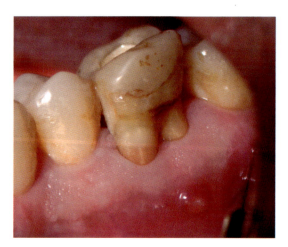

**Figure 2.33**

This mandibular molar presented with a buccal sinus tract and significant gingival recession exposing the furcation. An access cavity has been cut in the occlusal surface; however, the root canals had not been located.

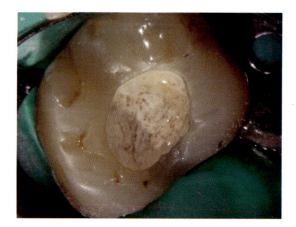

**Figure 2.34**

Under microscopic magnification, the temporary filling material in the access cavity was removed.

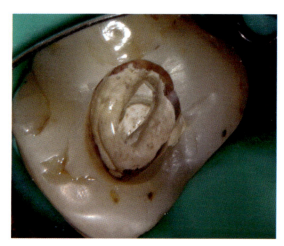

**Figure 2.35**

Using a bur, the superficial filling material was removed and the remainder carefully retrieved using ultrasonic tips.

approach to avoid the demise of new restorations. They may be better off with an alternative to complex root canal retreatment. Since root canal retreatment is often time-consuming, requiring dismantling of previous restorations and the removal of root-filling material before disinfecting the root canal system, it is important to make an assessment of the restorability of a tooth prior to embarking on prolonged and often expensive treatment. Alternatives to root canal retreatment, such as the placement of

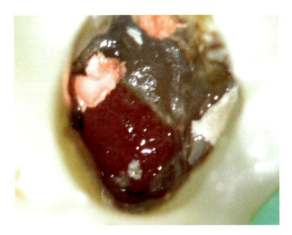

**Figure 2.36**

A view of the pulp floor unfortunately showed a large perforation. Hyperplastic gingival tissue had extended through the defect. The perforation site encompassed one of the root canals and the defect would therefore have been extremely difficult to seal. As there is direct communication between the pulp chamber and the furcation region of the tooth, coronal leakage and reinfection could be possible. Therefore, the prognosis for successful retreatment in this tooth was considered poor and it was extracted.

a fixed prosthesis or perhaps an implant-supported restoration, may offer a better long-term prognosis and should be considered at the treatment planning stage.

It has been reported that the quality of restoration and coronal seal may influence the outcome of endodontic treatment[29,30] and it is considered likely that many failures result from coronal microleakage. The ability of a well-prepared and filled root canal to resist frank and long-standing exposure by caries, fracture or loss of restoration may be considerably better than first thought.[31,32]

## Periodontal Assessment

During clinical assessment, a clear distinction needs to be made between periodontal pocketing that results from marginal periodontitis and that which occurs when a tooth is cracked or has a discharging sinus tract in the periodontal ligament space.

Teeth that have combined periodontic–endodontic problems will need combined treatment and it may be necessary to seek the opinion of a periodontist if a tooth appears to be severely compromised. The tooth should be viewed with regard to general oral health and, in some cases, extraction may be the best option.

## Patient Expectation

The patient should be included in the decision-making process. Following an explanation of the problem, possible treatment options, disease risk and likely cost of alternatives, the patient may decide not to have treatment. The patient's wishes must be respected as, medicolegally, patients must give consent to treatment before it starts. The final decision should be recorded with the clinician's advice.

Sometimes, patients' expectations can be unrealistic. They may be desperate to save a tooth that has an extremely poor prognosis and that should really be extracted. It is often unwise to embark on treatment in this case, as the problems only become compounded when things start to fail.

If patient expectations are commensurate with the clinician's expectations and experience, then a happy outcome should be achieved.

## Cost

Although a clinician will endeavour to avoid the removal of any functional natural tooth, this may not be an option because alternative treatment is too costly. The cost–benefit ratio of any treatment has to be weighed against all the alternative options.

Root canal retreatment and a new crown may be less expensive than the replacement of a tooth with a bridge or implant. Addition to an existing denture may be more cost-effective than complex root canal retreatment. It can be a difficult ethical dilemma to balance, but cost is an inevitable factor of modern dental practice.

## Risk

There are many potential risks involved in carrying out root canal retreatment. For example, there is the potential to damage an existing restoration when access is made through it. The patient will need to be informed that a new restoration could be required. Iatrogenic errors could occur during the process of removing the previous root-filling material or the root canal wall could be perforated while attempting to remove a fractured instrument. The clinician weighs up the risk of doing nothing, and therefore the potential of further pathology or pain, against the likelihood of achieving a better result and healing of an endodontic lesion.

Because non-surgical root canal retreatment is better able to eliminate root canal infection, is minimally invasive compared with surgery and is associated with fewer postoperative complications, the risk–benefit ratio would appear to favour a non-surgical approach. For these reasons, root canal retreatment is normally considered the primary approach for post-treatment disease.[33]

## TREATMENT PLANNING

Following the decision-making process, no active treatment or review may be considered appropriate. The incidence of the possibility of acute exacerbation per year from teeth with chronic apical periodontitis has been estimated as 5%. In other words, over a 10-year period 50% will flare up.[34] In cases where there is little or no periapical pathology present and the root filling is deficient but there are no clinical signs or symptoms, monitoring appears to result in complications in only a small percentage of cases.[19] Not providing treatment is only appropriate if there is a good coronal restoration, and the patient is aware of the potential risk of acute exacerbation.

General patient attitudes will influence treatment planning. The motivation to retain teeth, to pursue the best long-term treatment option and to spend time and money will vary between patients. This may be a primary consideration in the treatment planning process. For example, if a patient is not motivated to save teeth, extraction may be appropriate. If patients are aware that non-surgical treatment

will offer the best long-term prognosis but cannot devote sufficient time or have financial concerns, they may accept a surgical approach or extraction.[33]

Once a decision has been made to carry out retreatment, the clinician must decide whether a surgical, non-surgical or combined approach is most appropriate. The chance of teeth with no periapical pathology remaining symptom-free following root canal treatment or non-surgical retreatment has been shown to be 92–98%. When evidence of apical periodontitis is present, this is reduced to 74–86%. The chance of the teeth remaining functional is 91–97%. For root end surgery, the chance of teeth healing has been cited as an average of 70% and remaining functional as 86–92%.[35] Conservative endodontic therapy, both non-surgical and surgical, is therefore definitely justified and should be attempted when a good restorative and periodontal prognosis is projected, unless the patient is not motivated to retain the tooth. There is little evidence in the literature to recommend a surgical approach over a non-surgical approach, and the long-term success rates for surgical endodontics appear to be no better than a conventional approach.[36] But, surgical intervention is a far more radical procedure, generally demanding more expertise and resulting in a shortening of the clinical root length. As discussed in Chapter 1, the majority of endodontic failures occur as a result of infection within the root canal system. It is a futile exercise to attempt to incarcerate these organisms by carrying out root end surgery and placing an 'apical seal'. Unless the reservoir of infection is eliminated, it is likely to continue causing persistent periapical inflammation or failure of treatment. A surgical approach is normally reserved for situations in which, despite a good attempt at non-surgical retreatment, the tooth still presents with signs and symptoms (Figure 2.37).

## CONCLUSION

The consensus would therefore suggest that non-surgical root canal retreatment is often the most appropriate means of treating

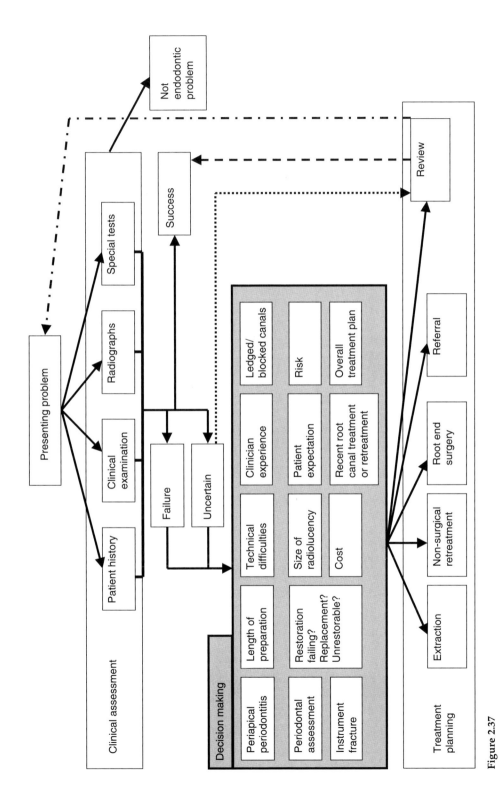

**Figure 2.37**

Root canal retreatment decision-making tree.

failed root-filled teeth in the first instance and that teeth should be permanently restored soon after retreatment to increase the chance of success.[37]

## REFERENCES

1. Strindberg LZ. The dependence of the results of pulp therapy on certain factors. *Acta Odontologica Scandinavica* 1956; **14**: (Suppl 21): 1–175.
2. European Society of Endodontology Concensus report of the European Society of Endodontology on quality guidelines for endodontic treatment. *International Endodontic Journal* 1994; **27**: 115–124.
3. Reit C. Decision strategies in endodontics: on the design of a recall program. *Endodontics and Dental Traumatology* 1987; **3**: 233–239.
4. Smith J, Crisp J, Torney D. A survey: controversies in endodontic treatment and retreatment. *Journal of Endodontics* 1981; **7**: 477–483.
5. Reit C, Gröndahl H-G. Management of periapical lesions in endodontically treated teeth. A study on clinical decision making. *Swedish Dental Journal* 1984; **8**: 1–7.
6. Reit C, Gröndahl H-G, Engström B. Endodontic treatment decisions: a study of the clinical decision-making process. *Endodontics and Dental Traumatology* 1985; **1**: 102–107.
7. Reit C, Gröndahl H-G. Endodontic retreatment decision making among a group of general practitioners. *Scandinavian Journal of Dental Research* 1988; **96**: 112–117.
8. Kvist T, Reit C, Esposito M, Mileman P, Bianchi S, Pettersson K, et al. Prescribing endodontic retreatment: towards a theory of dentist behaviour. *International Endodontic Journal* 1994; **27**: 285–290.
9. Kay E, Nuttall N. Clinical decision-making an art or a science? Part II making sense of treatment decisions. *British Dental Journal* 1995; **178**: 113–116.
10. Buckley GB, West B. A safe path or a legal minefield? *Health Bulletin* 1998; **56**: 848.
11. Bergenholtz G, Lekholm U, Milthon R, Heden G, Odesjo B, Engstrom B. Retreatment of endodontic fillings.

12. Eriksen H, Bjertness E. Prevalence of apical periodontitis and results of endodontic treatment in middle-aged adults in Norway. *Endodontics and Dental Traumatology* 1991; **7**: 1–4.
13. Eckerbom M, Anderson JE, Magnasson T. Frequency and technical standard of endodontic treatment in a Swedish population. *Endodontics and Dental Traumatology* 1987; **3**: 245–248.
14. Debelian GJ, Olsen I, Tronstad L. Systemic disease caused by oral microorganisms. *Endodontics and Dental Traumatology* 1994; **10**: 57–65.
15. Murray CA, Saunders WP. Root canal treatment and general health. A review of the literature. *International Endodontic Journal* 2000; **33**: 1–18.
16. Ørstavik D. Time-course and risk analyses of the development and healing of chronic apical periodontitis in man. *International Endodontic Journal* 1996; **29**: 150–155.
17. Ørstavik D, Kerekes K, Eriksen HM. The periapical index: a scoring system for radiographic assessment of apical periodontitis. *Endodontics and Dental Traumatology* 1986; **2**: 20–34.
18. Molven O, Halse A. Success rates for gutta percha and Kloropercha N-Ø root fillings made by undergraduate students: radiographic findings after 10–17 years. *International Endodontic Journal* 1988; **21**: 384–390.
19. Sjögren U, Häglund B, Sundqvist G, Wing K. Factors affecting the long-term results of endodontic treatment. *Journal of Endodontics* 1990; **16**: 498–504.
20. Friedman S, Löst C, Zarribian M, Trope M. Evaluation of success and failure after endodontic therapy using glass ionomer cement sealer. *Journal of Endodontics* 1995; **21**: 384–390.
21. Bergenholtz G, Lekholm U, Milthon R, Heden G, Ödesjö B, Engström B. Retreatment of endodontic fillings. *Scandinavian Journal of Dental Research* 1979; **87**: 217–224.
22. Van Nieuwenhuysen JP, Aouar M, D'Hoore W. Retreatment or radiographic monitoring in endodontics. *International Endodontic Journal* 1994; **27**: 75–81.

23. Bergenholtz G, Malmcrona E, Milthon R. Endodontic retreatment and periapical state. I Radiographic study of frequency of endodontically treated teeth and frequency of periapical lesions. *Tandlakartidningen* 1973; **65**: 64–73.

24. Chugal NM, Clive JM, Spangberg LS. Endodontic infection: some biologic and treatment factors associated with outcome. *Oral Surgey, Oral Medicine, Oral Pathology, Oral Radiology and Endodontics* 2003; **96**: 81–90.

25. Gorni FGM, Gagliani MM. The outcome of endodontic retreatment: a 2 yr follow-up. *Journal of Endodontics* 2004; **30**: 1–4.

26. Åkerblom A, Hasselgren G. The prognosis for endodontic treatment of obliterated root canals. *Journal of Endodontics* 1988; **14**: 565–567.

27. Hoskinson SE, Ng YL, Hoskinson AE, Moles DR, Gulabivala K. A retrospective comparison of outcome of root canal treatment using two different protocols. *Oral Surgery, Oral Medicine, Oral Pathology, Oral Radiology and Endodontics* 2002; **93**: 705–715.

28. Pitt Ford TR, Torabinejad T, McKendry DJ, Hong CU, Kariyawasam SP. Use of Mineral Trioxide Aggregate for repair of furcal perforations. *Oral Surgery, Oral Medicine, Oral Pathology, Oral Radiology and Endodontics* 1995; **79**: 756–762.

29. Ray HA, Trope M. Periapical status of endodontically treated teeth in relation to the technical quality of the root filling and the coronal restoration. *International Endodontic Journal* 1995; **28**: 12–18.

30. Saunders WP, Saunders EM. Coronal leakage as a cause of failure in root canal therapy: a review. *Endodontics and Dental Traumatology* 1994; **10**: 105–108.

31. Ricucci D, Bergenholtz G. Bacterial status in root-filled teeth exposed to the oral environment by loss of restoration and fracture or caries – a histobacteriological study of treated cases. *International Endodontic Journal* 2003; **36**: 787–802.

32. Torabinejad M, Ung B, Kettering JD. In vitro bacterial penetration of coronally unsealed endodontically treated teeth. *Journal of Endodontics* 1990; **16**: 566–569.

33. Friedman S. Considerations and concepts of case selection in the management of post-treatment endodontic disease (treatment failure). *Endodontic Topics* 2002; **1**: 54–78.

34. Eriksen H. Epidemiology of apical periodontitis. In: Ørstavik D, Pitt Ford TR, eds. *Essential endodontology* Oxford: Blackwell Science; 1998.

35. Friedman S, Mor C. The success of endodontic therapy – healing and functionality. *Journal of Californian Dental Association* 2004; **32**: 493–503.

36. Friedman S. Treatment outcome and prognosis of endodontic therapy. In: Ørstavik D, Pitt Ford TR, eds. *Essential endodontology*. Oxford: Blackwell Science; 1998.

37. Briggs PFA, Scott BJJ. Evidenced-based dentistry: endodontic failure – how should it be managed? *British Dental Journal* 1997; **183**: 159–164.

# 3 DISMANTLING CORONAL RESTORATIONS

**CONTENTS** • Introduction • Removing Crowns • Methods for Removing Crowns • Removal of Posts • Removing Plastic Core Material • References

## INTRODUCTION

Gaining access to root canals for non-surgical retreatment is relatively easy when a direct intracoronal restoration is in place. However, dismantling cast restorations, posts and cores can be challenging. The techniques described in this chapter will allow predictable disassembly for non-surgical root canal retreatment.

## REMOVING CROWNS

It is not uncommon for a crown to be removed in order to complete root canal retreatment. It is therefore always wise to warn a patient that a new restoration may be required before embarking on dismantling the root-treated tooth. Patients are more likely to accept the potential additional cost of a new restoration if they have been advised that the existing one may be damaged or destroyed in the process of root canal retreatment.

The quality of coronal seal should be assessed preoperatively. Where a crown is obviously leaking or has been undermined by recurrent caries, it should be removed. Removing the coronal restoration will obviously give much better information about the state of the remaining tooth substance. There is little justification in attempting to retain an existing restoration if it is going to jeopardize successful root canal retreatment. Removing the coronal restoration may also be important in deciding whether a tooth is actually restorable. After all, unless the foundation work can be completed successfully, extraction may

be the only course of action. Removing a restoration, therefore, allows thorough investigation, assessment of restorability, removal of caries and location of orifices which may not be possible when working through an access cavity. Difficulty in locating canals can be especially relevant if the crown does not conform to the original anatomy of the tooth, thereby giving a false indication of where the canal orifices may lie (Figure 3.1).[1]

From a technical viewpoint, it can sometimes be difficult to achieve good positioning of the rubber dam clamp when a crown has been removed. In this case it may be recemented as

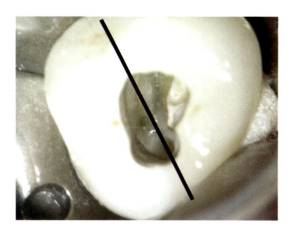

**Figure 3.1**

The bonded metal ceramic crown on this maxillary molar is orientated such that the occlusal surface is rotated in respect to the underlying tooth substance. The mesiobuccal canal now lies in the midline. It is easy to lose direction when cutting access cavities through bonded restorations. The pulp floor map should be used to highlight the orifices of canals. Generally, the pulp floor is darker than the walls.

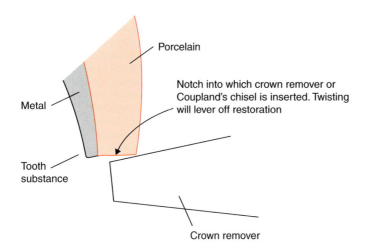

**Figure 3.2**

Removal of crowns.

a temporary measure with glass ionomer following caries removal[2] or a temporary restoration may be constructed. Alternatively, a split dam technique may be required. If there is insufficient tooth substance remaining onto which a rubber dam clamp can be placed, then one must question whether the tooth is actually restorable. If the crown is of good quality and has only recently been fitted, root canal retreatment can normally be carried out through a conservative access cavity which will be sealed using adhesive restorative materials following treatment.

## METHODS FOR REMOVING CROWNS

### Chisel, Flat Plastic and Coupland's Chisel

Careful placement of a chisel, flat plastic or Coupland's chisel into a marginal deficiency can be sufficient to cause the cement lute to fail. Force should be applied along the path of insertion to avoid fracture of the underlying tooth substance and core material. The chisel should be held in the palm of the hand with the forefinger near the tip so that if the instrument slips there is no risk of injury to the patient. The margin of the crown can be undermined using a small diamond bur or an

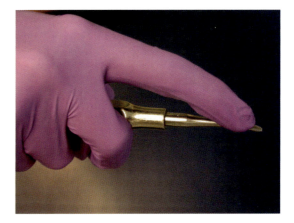

**Figure 3.3**

A Coupland's chisel should be held firmly in the hand with a forefinger placed near the blade. This will help prevent injury to the patient should the instrument slip.

ultrasonic tip, creating a gap into which the chisel is placed (Figures 3.2–3.5).

An access cavity can be cut in the occlusal surface and the instrument inserted between underlying core material and the crown. By cutting an access cavity, retention of the crown is significantly reduced and should therefore make crown removal easier. There are numerous burs available for preparing an occlusal cavity through crowns. Usually, a diamond bur is preferred for cutting porcelain and a

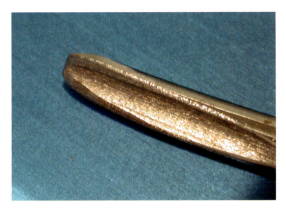

**Figure 3.4**

The tip of the Coupland's chisel has been modified for use in removing cast restorations.

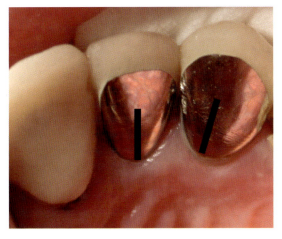

**Figure 3.5**

When removing anterior crowns, it is sometimes possible to cut a groove in the palatal aspect of the crown (as shown by the black lines) into which a flat plastic or Coupland's chisel can be inserted. Flexing the crown allows removal so that the restoration may be recemented as a temporary.

tungsten carbide bur used to cut through the metal part of any restoration.

## *Forceps*

Special forceps for crown removal are available with rubber cups on the beaks. These are coated in carborundum powder to prevent slipping. Some practitioners prefer to use extraction

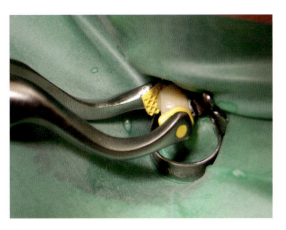

**Figure 3.6**

Specialist crown pliers can be used to remove restorations.

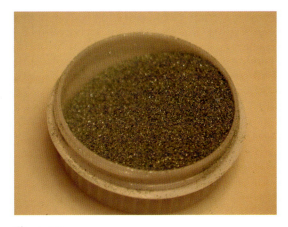

**Figure 3.7**

The rubber beaks of the pliers are coated in carborundum powder to improve the grip.

forceps, but great care must be exercised to ensure that the instrument does not slip or that excessive force is placed on the tooth, thereby damaging it. Generally, forceps are applied to the crown that needs to be removed and a gentle wiggling action used to loosen the restoration. One must be careful not to damage adjacent or opposing teeth (Figures 3.6, 3.7).

## *The Richwell Crown and Bridge Remover*

This is essentially a tablet of water-soluble pliable resin which is softened in hot water and placed on the restoration that needs to be removed. The patient is asked to bite down and compress the resin block to about two-thirds of its original thickness. It is then allowed to cool. When the resin is set, the patient is asked to open quickly, which, in theory, will generate sufficient force to loosen and lift the restoration. This technique tends not to be particularly effective. There is also a risk of removing the restoration from an opposing tooth!

## Ultrasonics

Ultrasonics is sometimes useful to loosen the cement from around the margins of a poorly fitting crown. This could be a simple ultrasonic scaler tip vibrated at high power with a water spray or a specialist tip such as the CT4 (SybronEndo, Orange, CA, USA). If a porcelain crown needs to be removed with little damage, then ultrasonics should not be used as there is the potential risk of porcelain fracture. Undermining the crown or opening up a marginal deficiency will allow the placement of a crown remover, chisel or flat plastic (Figure 3.8).

## Chisel and Mallet

A straight chisel and mallet can be used to tap off the crown. However, there are obvious risks involved in this method and it is perhaps not that pleasant for the patient!

## Crown Removers

This instrument consists of a hook that is inserted under the margin of a restoration. The hook is in turn connected to a rod with either a weight or a spring-loaded device which can apply a sudden force to break the cement lute. Well-fitting restorations obviously present a problem, as it is difficult to find a margin under which the instrument can be inserted. The KaVo Coronaflex (KaVo Dental Ltd, Amersham, Buckinghamshire, UK) works by delivering a pneumatic force. Special forceps or bands are provided which can be linked to either crowns or bridges. On depressing the trigger, a force is generated along the long access of the tooth, enabling removal of the restoration. This is an excellent device for removing restorations with little risk of damage (Figures 3.9–3.13).

## The WamKey

The WamKey (Dentsply, Weybridge, Surrey, UK) looks rather like a small key and can be

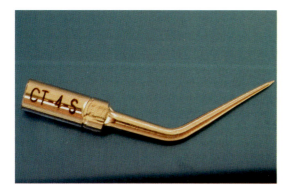

**Figure 3.8**

A CT4 tip can be used to remove cement from around the margins of a cast restoration.

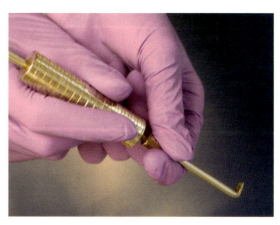

**Figure 3.9**

A crown tapper can be used to remove cast restorations. The beak of the instrument is placed underneath the crown margin and the weights used to produce a sudden force in the long access of the tooth.

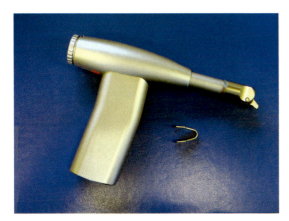

**Figure 3.10**

The KaVo CORONAflex pneumatic crown and bridge remover.

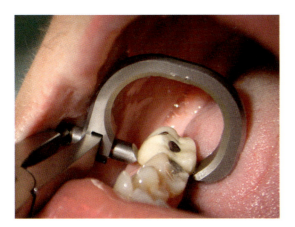

**Figure 3.11**

The KaVo CORONAflex forceps are placed at the margins of the restoration.

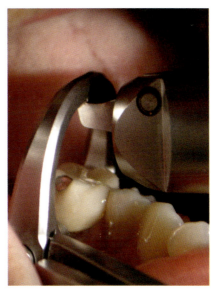

**Figure 3.12**

The pneumatic handpiece is used to deliver a sudden force into the hoop of the forceps.

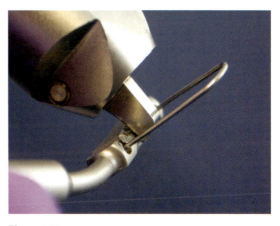

**Figure 3.13**

A wire loop is inserted under the pontic of a bridge for removal with this device.

effective for crown and bridge removal. A small access is cut in the buccal or lingual surface of the crown such that space is made between the underside of the restoration and any core material. The key is then inserted and, when rotated, separates the crown from the underlying core material (Figures 3.14–3.17).

## Sectioning

If a crown is to be replaced, it can simply be removed by sectioning with a bur and the separate pieces elevated. Metal restorations can easily be cut using a tungsten carbide fissure bur such as a Jet Beaver bur (Beavers Dental, Morrisburg, Ontario, Canada).[3]

The crown is partially sectioned by cutting a groove from the gingival to the occlusal surface and then a crown remover, flat plastic or Coupland's chisel can be used to open up the

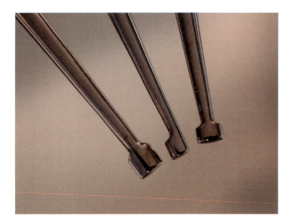

**Figure 3.14**

The heads of the WamKeys.

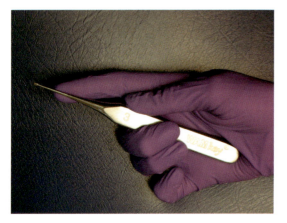

**Figure 3.15**

The WamKey is grasped in the palm of the hand and a twisting action used to break the cement lute.

groove and flex the restoration, breaking the cement lute. One should make sure that the restoration has been completely severed at the gingival margin. Some crowns, if particularly well cemented, will need to be 'peeled' off the tooth. Cutting a slot and prizing the crown loose is probably the least traumatic method of removing a cast restoration. Even though the crown may be destroyed, damage to the tooth is avoided (Figures 3.18, 3.19).[4]

## Bridges

The abutment teeth of bridges can normally be treated as individual crowns and access is

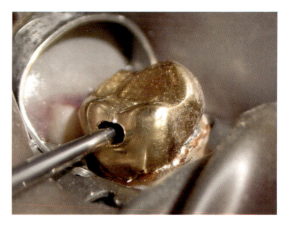

**Figure 3.16**

A small access has been cut in the buccal surface of this full-coverage gold crown. The WamKey has been inserted into it and, when rotated, directs force between the underside of the crown and the core material.

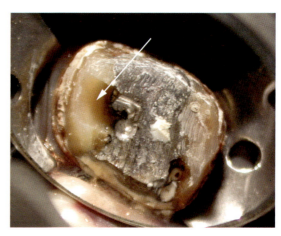

**Figure 3.17**

The crown has been removed and the 'letterbox' access can be seen on the buccal aspect. In this case the restoration was recemented as a temporary.

often made in the occlusal surface in the normal manner. A split dam technique can be useful to gain isolation and caulking will be required to block out the area under pontics.[2] If the bridge is to be sectioned and removed, it is important that the remaining portion, if cantilevered, does not allow excessive force to be placed on the abutment so risking fracture. In the anterior region of the mouth where aesthetics are important, it may be easier and beneficial to construct a temporary bridge

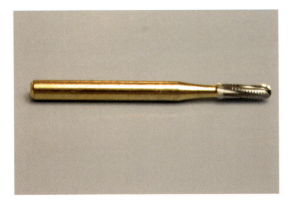

**Figure 3.18**

A tungsten carbide fissure bur is very effective for sectioning metal restorations.

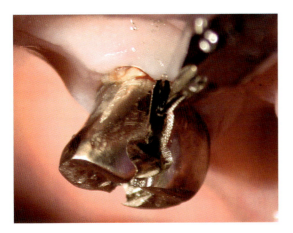

**Figure 3.19**

This crown could not be removed using a WamKey and it has therefore been sectioned. A crown-removing tool has been inserted into the groove and, on rotation, will separate the two halves.

using an acrylic material. When glazed and polished a very good cosmetic result can be achieved. Alternatively, a temporary denture may be provided (Figure 3.20).

## REMOVAL OF POSTS

Post removal has been shown to be a predictable procedure, and using appropriate techniques rarely results in root fracture.[5]

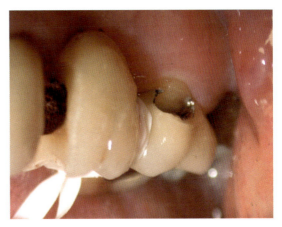

**Figure 3.20**

A bridge has been sectioned. Before removal, floss is tied to the pontic. This prevents the risk of swallowing it should the distal portion become dislodged. A small groove has been cut at the margin of the distal abutment into which a chisel can be inserted for removal.

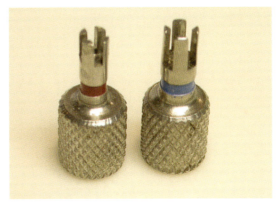

**Figure 3.21**

Radix Anker wrenches can be used to remove their corresponding posts.

### Screw Posts

The simplest means of removing a screw post is to use the wrench provided by the manufacturer for insertion (Figures 3.21, 3.22).

Core material is carefully removed from around the post using a bur and ultrasonic tips such as the CT4, CPR 2 (Obtura Spartan Corp., Fenton, MO, USA), BUC-1 (Obtura Spartan Corp., Fenton, MO, USA), or Pro-Ultra Endo tips 2 or 3 (Dentsply-Maillefer, Ballaigues,

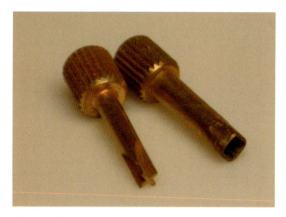

**Figure 3.22**

Dentatus screw-posts come with two wrenches: a cross-head, which can be used to slot into the head of the Dentatus screw; and a box wrench, which can be fitted over the head.

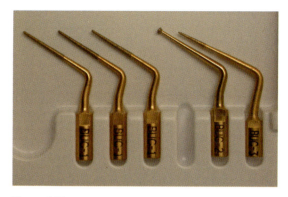

**Figure 3.24**

The BUC tips.

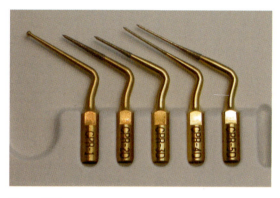

**Figure 3.23**

The CPR range of ultrasonic tips. The CPR 1 is for post removal. Tips 2 to 5 are all diamond coated and can be used at varying depths within the root canal.

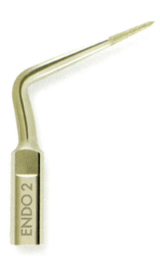

**Figure 3.25**

A Pro-Ultra Tip 2.

Switzerland). The head of the post remains intact. Ultrasonic tips are used in a Pieson ultrasonic unit and vibrated at reasonably high force with water spray. Both Cavitron and Pieson units have been shown to be useful in post removal but sonic devices are not effective.[6] It may sometimes be necessary to remove some of the cement lute with ultrasonics prior to using a wrench. The Dentatus (Dentatus AB, Hägersten, Sweden) or Radix Anker (Dentsply, Weybridge, Surrey, UK) are two types of screw posts (Figures 3.23–3.27).

The Radix Anker has grooves along the main shaft into which material can become locked. Care should be exercised when attempting to remove such a post and the wrench should never be forced (Figures 3.28–3.30).

Following core removal and undermining of the cement from around a post, the corresponding wrench is fitted to the head of the post and unscrewed. If the head of the post has been damaged and the wrench no longer fits, then a small piece of cotton wool can simply be placed over the end of the post, and the wrench wedged onto it before removal.

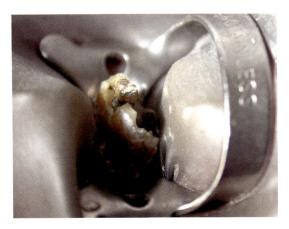

**Figure 3.26**

This tooth has been restored using a Dentatus post and amalgam core. The core material has been removed with ultrasonics and the head of the Dentatus post is now uncovered.

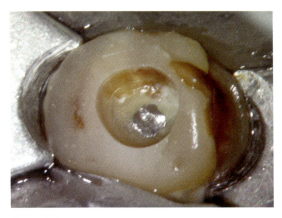

**Figure 3.28**

In this case a well-cemented Radix Anker post has been used to build up the tooth. The head of the post is uncovered using diamond high-speed burs.

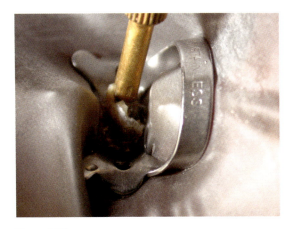

**Figure 3.27**

The box wrench is placed over the head of the Dentatus post and rotated anticlockwise to remove it.

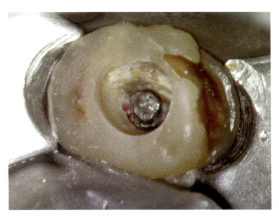

**Figure 3.29**

The cement around the post can then be undermined with ultrasonic tips. The Radix Anker has grooves along the shank and cement will need to be removed from these in order to allow the post to be retrieved.

Screw posts can sometimes be removed using ultrasound. The ultrasonic tip is worked around the post in an anticlockwise direction to help loosen and unscrew it. If it is sufficiently loose, the post may actually unwind itself from the root canal. Ultrasonic vibration is one of the most common methods used to remove posts and rarely results in root fracture.[7]

## Cast Posts

Cast posts are commonly used to restore anterior teeth. More complex cast cores are sometimes found on posterior teeth and can be dismantled using similar methods. If there is post retention in more than one canal in a posterior tooth, it is prudent to section the core material into individual pieces using a tungsten carbide bur before attempting removal.

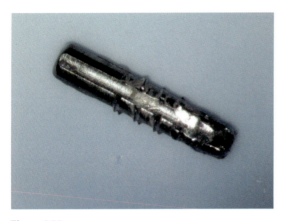

**Figure 3.30**

The Radix Anker showing the groove along its shank. If this is filled with resin-based cement, removal can be more difficult.

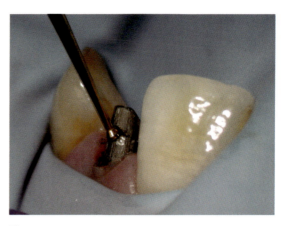

**Figure 3.32**

A notch is cut in the cast core into which the CPR 1 tip can be placed. This allows ultrasonic vibration to be applied in the long access of the tooth.

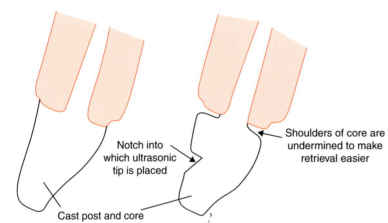

**Figure 3.31**

Removal of cast post with ultrasonics.

There are three phases to the removal of a cast post (Figures 3.31–3.42):

- Removal of the coronal restoration – having decided on the form of temporary restoration, the coronal restoration covering the post and core is removed.
- Uncovering the post – any remaining restorative material covering the post will need to be removed using ultrasonics.
- Extraction – a small rest seat is cut into the core material in which the ultrasonic tip can be inserted. Ultrasonic force is applied in the long access of the tooth to help loosen the cement. A thick ultrasonic scaler tip or CPR 1 should be used to efficiently transmit ultrasonic power to the post. If the post is

not completely removed with ultrasonic vibration after a period of 10–15 minutes, an alternative method would be used and less force should subsequently be required.[8] It is sometimes helpful to undermine the margins of the core material to aid removal. This can be achieved either with an ultrasonic tip or LN bur (B205 LN bur, Dentsply-Maillefer, Ballaigues, Switzerland).

## Post Removal Devices

There are several post removal devices available including the Sword post puller (Carl Martin GmbH, Solingen, Germany), the Eggler post remover (Automaton-Vertriebs-Gesellschaft,

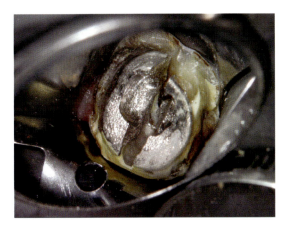

**Figure 3.33**

When removing a complex posterior cast core, material is normally sectioned into pieces before removal. In this case the mandibular molar has been restored with a cast core. The core has been sectioned into two halves using a tungsten carbide fissure bur.

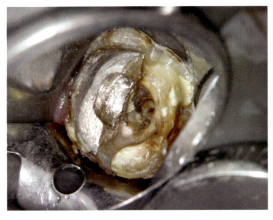

**Figure 3.34**

The distal portion was removed using ultrasonics.

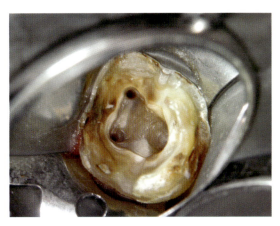

**Figure 3.35**

The mesial portion was then retrieved and debris and caries removed from the coronal tooth substance prior to root canal retreatment.

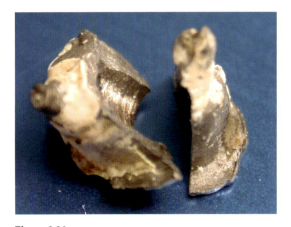

**Figure 3.36**

The pieces of core material as removed.

Germany),[9] the Gonon or Thomas post remover[10] (FFDM-Pneumat, Bourges, France) and the Ruddle post removal system (SybronEndo, Orange, CA, USA). Essentially all these devices work on the principle of exerting a force between the root face and the post such that the cement lute can be broken. Once this has been achieved, the post can easily be removed with Stieglitz forceps. Although post removers have been shown to be more efficient in removing posts,[11] vibration with ultrasound does significantly decrease the force required for removal.[12] Post removers should never be used to try removing screw-type posts.

*The Ruddle Post Removal Kit*
The core material must first be reduced in size so that a trephine drill can be used to mill the core into a cylinder. Several rubber bungs that will rest on the root surface and protect it are fitted onto the shaft of the remover. This is then screwed onto the milled core and the jaws of the extracting pliers placed between the head of the tap and the rubber bungs.

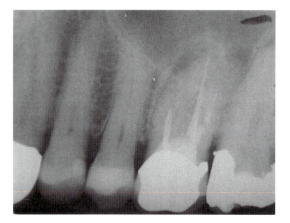

**Figure 3.37**

This maxillary left first molar has been restored with a composite core and has a titanium post in the distobuccal canal. The crown is of good quality and appears to have no marginal defects. The root filling is short in the mesiobuccal canal and there is a periapical radiolucency present.

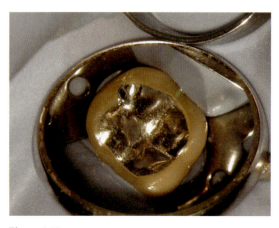

**Figure 3.38**

It was decided to carry out root canal retreatment and retain the existing crown. Access was cut through the metal occlusal surface.

When opened by rotating a screw, force is exerted along the long axis of the post and causes the cement lute to fail (Figures 3.43–3.52).

*The Sword Post Puller*

This is a neat little device with jaws that grip the head of the post and feet that fit on the shoulders of the root surface. As the screw is

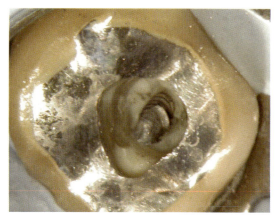

**Figure 3.39**

Using a tungsten carbide fissure bur, the head of the titanium post was uncovered and some of the composite core material removed.

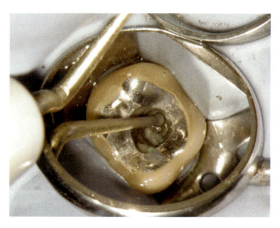

**Figure 3.40**

A diamond-coated ultrasonic tip was used to remove core material from around the post. A CPR 1 tip was then used to vibrate the post until the cement lute failed.

tightened, forces are exerted along the length of the post, breaking the cement lute (Figure 3.53).

Post Fracture with no Supracoronal Material Remaining

When the post has fractured within the root canal, a remover will be required in order to retrieve the fractured segment. There are three

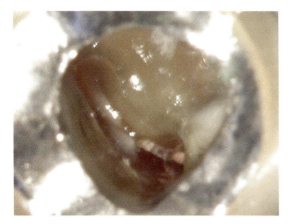

**Figure 3.41**

Following removal, the pulp floor was cleaned. There were two canals in the mesiobuccal root. There is some gutta percha retained in a fin adjacent to the main mesiobuccal canal. The second mesiobuccal canal had not been prepared during primary treatment. This highlights the importance of using a solvent when removing condensed gutta percha from root-treated teeth.

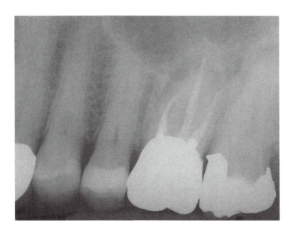

**Figure 3.42**

The completed case. Four root canals have been thoroughly cleaned and, following medication, obturated using a vertically compacted gutta percha technique. The access cavity has been sealed by the placement of a Nayyar core.

phases to the removal of fractured posts from within the root canal system:

- Make space – space is required to allow removal of the fractured piece of post. This provides an exit pathway.
- Loosen – the post fragment or post is normally loosened using ultrasonics. This

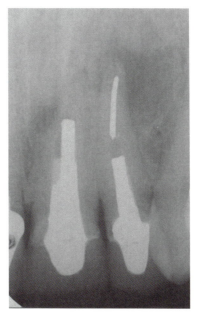

**Figure 3.43**

The maxillary central and lateral incisor teeth both have large posts in place. There is a large periapical radiolucency around the root ends. In order to eradicate intraradicular infection, non-surgical root canal retreatment would be required. Apical surgery in this instance would not be helpful as it would be extremely difficult to clean the root canal effectively. There may potentially be a root perforation on the maxillary left central incisor.

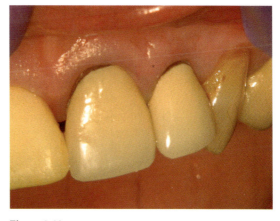

**Figure 3.44**

The crowns were easily removed by inserting a flat plastic under the margins.

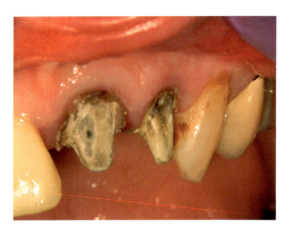

**Figure 3.45**

The cast cores were revealed.

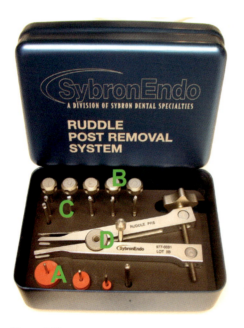

**Figure 3.46**

The Ruddle post removal kit is similar to the Gonon kit and consists of (A) rubber bungs to protect the tooth, (B) self-tapping removers, (C) trephine drills and (D) pliers.

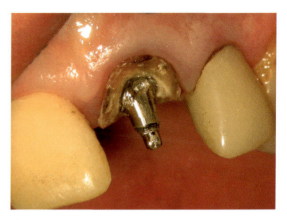

**Figure 3.47**

Using a tungsten carbide non-end cutting bur, core material was reduced so that a trephine from the Ruddle post removal kit could be fitted over it. The trephine machines the core material into a cylinder onto which a self-tapping remover can be fitted.

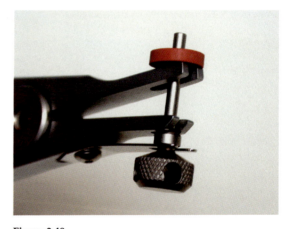

**Figure 3.48**

The removal assembly consisting of self-tapping remover, rubber bung and pliers.

*The Masserann Kit*
The Masserann kit is shown in Figure 3.54.

*Trephines*
The Masserann device (Micromega, Besancon, France) was designed for the removal of metallic objects lodged in the root canal. The kit consists of a series of 14 colour-coded trephines, ranging from 1.1 to 2.4 mm. The trephines are designed for removing material from around a fractured object, for gripping it

may take between 2 and 16 minutes.[13,14] Irrigant spray will also break up and remove luting cement from around the post.

- Removal/retrieval – if the post cannot be removed using ultrasonics alone, then it can usually be retrieved using the Masserann kit.

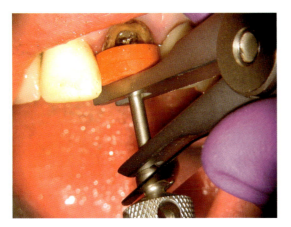

**Figure 3.49**

The self-tapping remover has been screwed onto the coronal part of the cast post. Rubber bungs are placed on the shoulders of the tooth and the jaws of the pliers connected.

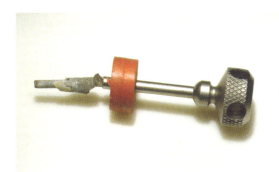

**Figure 3.50**

Once the cement lute has failed, the post is easily withdrawn.

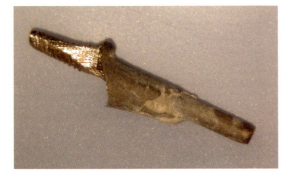

**Figure 3.51**

It is possible to see the screw thread that was tapped into the remaining core material.

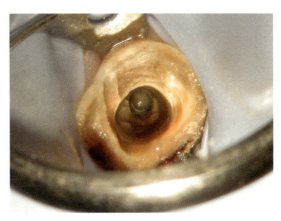

**Figure 3.52**

Looking down the root canal, retained cement is visible. This can easily be removed using a long, diamond-coated ultrasonic tip such as the CPR 4 or 5.

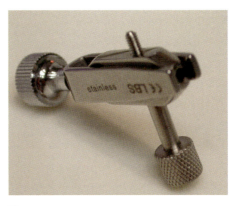

**Figure 3.53**

The sword post puller works in a similar way to other post removers. Two shoulders rest on the tooth substance while the beaks grip the post that has to be removed.

and extracting large-diameter objects such as posts.[15] This device is best used in the coronal aspect of the root canal, where access is good (Figure 3.55).

*Extractors*

Two extractors, consisting of a rod and tube, can be used for removing smaller-diameter objects such as silver points and instrument fragments. There are probably more conservative methods available for working within the confines of the root canal (Figure 3.56).

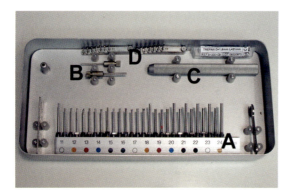

**Figure 3.54**

The Masserran kit consists of (A) a series of graded trephine drills, (B) Masserran removers for smaller objects, (C) a handle for attaching to the trephines and (D) a gauge.

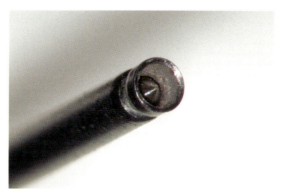

**Figure 3.56**

A Masserran remover is designed for the removal of smaller items. It consists of a tube into which a rod is inserted. The two are screwed together and grip the fragment that is to be retrieved.

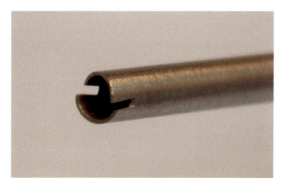

**Figure 3.55**

A Masserran trephine can be used to remove dentine from around a fractured post very conservatively. The blades work in an anticlockwise direction.

*Gauges*

There are two sets of gauges, which correspond to the trephines and can be used as measuring devices (Figure 3.57).

The trephines can be used in a speed-reducing handpiece or attached to a long handle that is rotated by hand. The trephines cut in an anticlockwise direction. If the post has a circular cross section, a trephine is selected that is very slightly larger than the post diameter. This is used to remove a very small amount of dentine and any cement lute from around the head of the fractured post. An ultrasonic tip such as a CT4, CPR 1 or scaler tip[16] can then be used to vibrate the post fragment. The unit is used at high power with irrigant spray. The

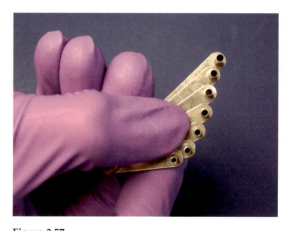

**Figure 3.57**

Gauges can be used to measure the size of fractured post.

irrigant spray helps to remove any cement lute as it is dislodged. The next size of trephine is then selected. This will grip the fragment of post in the root canal and can be used to retrieve it. The Masserann kit is an excellent means of removing fractured cylindrical post fragments from the coronal part of the root canal.

Removal will probably be more difficult if resin cements have been used to cement the post.[17,18] In the clinical environment, microleakage will often contribute to failure of the cement lute and subsequently help reduce the time required for removal (Figures 3.58–3.63).[19]

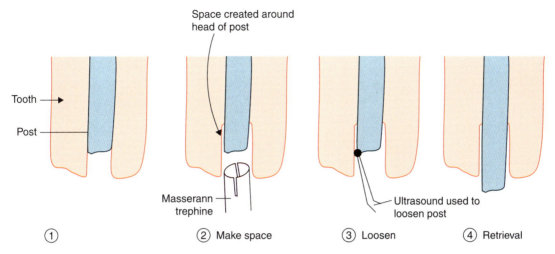

**Figure 3.58**

Removal of fractured post.

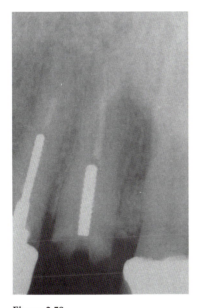

**Figure 3.59**

This radiograph shows a maxillary incisor in which a post has fractured. The tooth is restorable as there is sufficient tooth substance remaining to provide a ferrule. During removal, as much of the coronal tooth substance should be preserved as possible.

## Fibre Posts

Fibre posts are constructed of carbon fibre, glass or quartz fibres in a composite matrix.

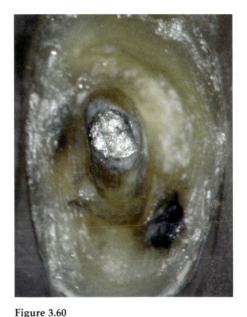

**Figure 3.60**

A fractured post viewed through an operating microscope.

They are normally bonded into the root canal using dentine bonding agents. This can sometimes make them difficult to remove. Fortunately, most of the posts that will need to be removed during root canal retreatment will have failed as a result of coronal microleakage and, therefore, the bond interface has often failed. These can sometimes be removed using

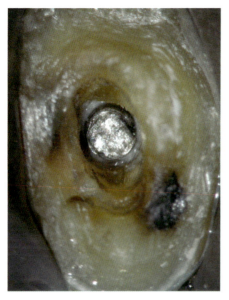

**Figure 3.61**

Cement and a small amount of dentine are removed using a Masserran trephine. This is far more conservative than using ultrasonics and does not risk perforation or gross damage that can occur with burs. It will be more difficult to remove posts that have been cemented with resin cements.

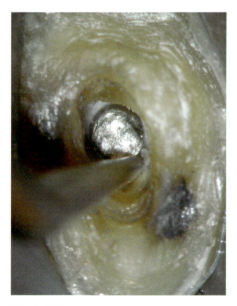

**Figure 3.62**

Once 2–4 mm of post have been uncovered, ultrasonics are used to loosen the post fragment.

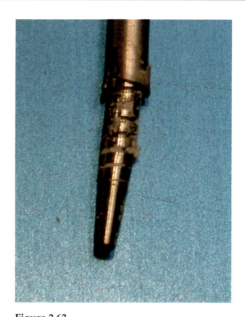

**Figure 3.63**

The post is then retrieved using a smaller Masserran trephine.

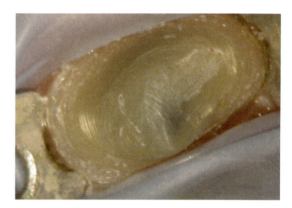

**Figure 3.64**

This tooth has been restored with a carbon fibre post and composite core.

artery forceps or a post puller. Well-cemented posts can be drilled out using special burs from the corresponding post removal kit.[20] A round swan neck bur (DT205 LN bur, Dentsply-Maillefer, Ballaigues, Switzerland) can be used to create a pilot channel down the centre of the post. The post can then be removed using Peeso drills, or Gates–Glidden burs. Finally, remaining fragments are removed using the proprietary post drill from the relevant post kit (Figures 3.64–3.68).

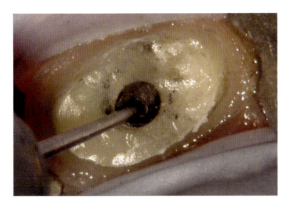

**Figure 3.65**

Composite is removed using a diamond bur to uncover the fibre post. The LN bur is used to make a pilot hole along the centre of the post.

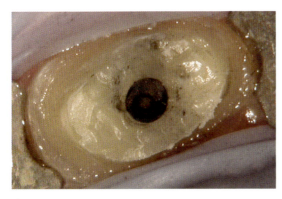

**Figure 3.66**

The pilot channel in the centre of the post.

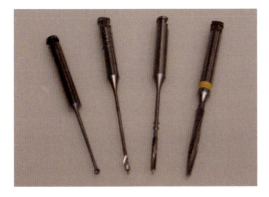

**Figure 3.67**

An LN bur, Gates–Glidden bur, Peeso drill and fibre post drill.

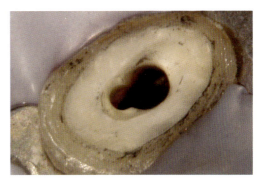

**Figure 3.68**

The remainder of the post was removed using a post drill.

## REMOVING PLASTIC CORE MATERIAL

Cores are generally constructed from amalgam or composite. The Nayyar core[21] is advocated as a means of restoring posterior teeth without the need for posts. The material is normally packed into the coronal 3 mm of the root canals. It is very important not to try removing this material using a bur, as the risk of root perforation is high.

### Dismantling a Nayyar Core

Using a paralleling radiograph, an estimate can be made of the depth of material to the level of the pulp floor. Using magnification, the coronal portion of the restoration is removed either with a tungsten carbide or diamond bur. The material is removed laterally until the boundaries of the pulp chamber become evident. The core material is then removed until the pulp floor just becomes visible. An ultrasonic tip such as a CT4, CPR 2, BUC-1 or Pro-Ultra Endo tip 2 is then used on medium to high power with irrigant spray to carefully remove core material across the pulp floor. Using the same instrument, material can be removed very conservatively from the coronal part of the root canal without risking perforation.[22] The CPR 2, BUC-1 and Pro-Ultra Endo 2 tips are coated with abrasive material, which aids removal of restorative materials in such a situation (Figures 3.69–3.78).

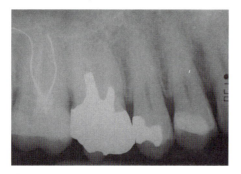

**Figure 3.69**

An amalgam Nayyar core has been constructed on this maxillary right first molar tooth. There is little evidence of root-filling material in the root canals and the palatal root has periapical pathology associated with it.

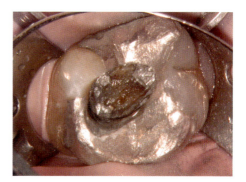

**Figure 3.72**

Eventually, the canal orifices, which were packed with amalgam, were located.

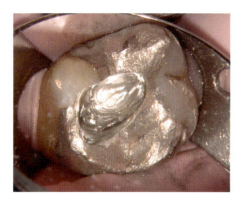

**Figure 3.70**

Core material was carefully removed from the coronal part of the tooth using a tungsten carbide fissure bur. The lateral boundaries of the previous access cavity were located.

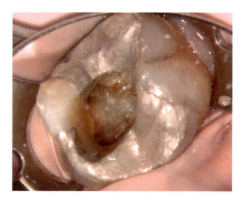

**Figure 3.73**

The amalgam was removed conservatively from them using the same ultrasonic tip.

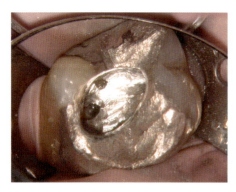

**Figure 3.71**

When the pulp floor was reached, a diamond-coated ultrasonic tip was used to break up material lying across the floor and retained on the walls.

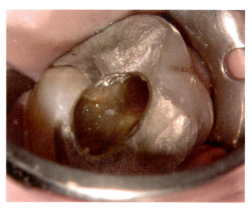

**Figure 3.74**

Following removal of the core, root canal retreatment could be completed.

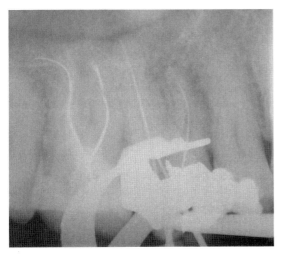

**Figure 3.75**

A diagnostic working length radiograph shows the canals renegotiated following removal of the core material.

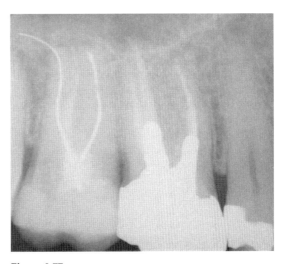

**Figure 3.77**

Three months later, a radiograph revealed evidence of healing. A sinus tract that was present before treatment had healed and the tooth was symptom-free.

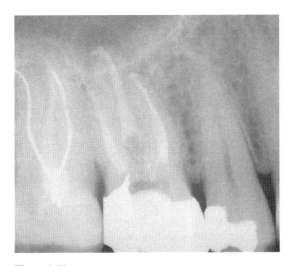

**Figure 3.76**

The case completed.

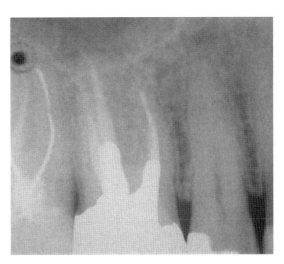

**Figure 3.78**

Six months following root canal retreatment, there appeared to be complete healing radiographically and the tooth will be restored with a cast restoration.

## REFERENCES

1. Parreira FR, O'Connor RP, Hutter JW. Cast prosthesis removal using ultrasonics and a thermoplastic resin adhesive. *Journal of Endodontics* 1994; **20**: 141–143.
2. Pitt Ford TR, Rhodes JS, Pitt Ford HE. *Endodontics: Problem-solving in clinical practice*. London: Martin Dunitz; 2002.
3. Siegel SC, Von Fraunhofer JA. Comparison of sectioning rates among carbide and diamond burs using three casting alloys. *Journal of Prosthodontics* 1999; **8**: 240–244.
4. Oliva RA. Review of methods for removing cast gold restorations. *Journal of*

*American Dental Association* 1979; **99**: 840–847.

5. Abbott PV. Incidence of root fractures and methods used for post removal. *International Endodontic Journal* 2002; **35**: 63–67.

6. Buoncristiani J, Seto BG, Caputo AA. Evaluation of ultrasonic and sonic instruments for intraradicular post removal. *Journal of Endodontics* 1994; **20**: 486–489.

7. Castrisos T, Abbott PV. A survey of methods used for post removal in specialist endodontic practice. *International Endodontic Journal* 2002; **35**: 172–180.

8. Berbert A, Filho MT, Ueno AH, Bramante CM, Ishikiriama A. The influence of ultrasound in removing intraradicular posts. *International Endodontic Journal* 1995; **28**: 100–102.

9. Castrisos T, Palamara JE, Abbott PV. Measurement of strain on tooth roots during post removal with the Eggler post remover. *International Endodontic Journal* 2002; **35**: 337–344.

10. Machtou P, Sarfati P, Cohen AG. Post removal prior to retreatment. *Journal of Endodontics* 1989; **15**: 552–554.

11. Altshul JH, Marshall G, Morgan LA, Baumgartner JC. Comparison of dentinal crack incidence and of post removal time resulting from post removal by ultrasonic or mechanical force. *Journal of Endodontics* 1997; **23**: 683–686.

12. Gomes AP, Kubo CH, Santos RA, Santos DR, Padiha RQ. The influence of ultrasound on the retention of cast posts cemented with different agents. *International Endodontic Journal* 2001; **34**: 93–99.

13. Dixon EB, Kaczkowski PJ, Nicholls JI, Harrington GW. Comparison of two ultrasonic units for post removal. *Journal of Endodontics* 2002; **28**: 111–115.

14. Johnson WT, Leary JM, Boyer DB. Effect of ultrasonic vibration on post removal in extracted human premolar teeth. *Journal of Endodontics* 1996; **22**: 487–488.

15. Williams VD, Bjorndal AM. The Masserann technique for the removal of fractured posts in endodontically treated teeth. *Journal of Prosthodontic Dentistry* 1983; **49**: 46–48.

16. Krell KV, Jordan RD, Madison S, Aquilino S. Using ultrasonic scalers to remove fractured root posts. *Journal of Prosthodontic Dentistry* 1986; **55**: 46–49.

17. Smith BJ. The removal of fractured post fragments in general dental practice using ultrasonic vibration. *Dental Update* 2002; **29**: 488–491.

18. Chandler NP, Qualtrough AJ, Purton DG. Comparison of two methods for the removal of root canal posts. *Quintessence International* 2003; **34**: 534–536.

19. Smith BJ. Removal of fractured posts using ultrasonic vibration: an in vivo study. *Journal of Endodontics* 2001; **27**: 632–634.

20. Gesi A, Magnolfi S, Gorracci C, Ferrari M. Comparison of two techniques for removing fibre posts. *Journal of Endodontics* 2003; **29**: 580–582.

21. Nayyar A, Walton RE, Leonard LA. An amalgam coronal-radicular dowel and core technique for endodontically treated posterior teeth. *Journal of Prosthetic Dentistry* 1980; **43**: 511–515.

22. Goon VW. Efficient amalgam core elimination and root preservation with ultrasonic instrumentation. *Journal of Prosthetic Dentistry* 1992; **68**: 261–264.

# 4 REMOVAL OF PASTES, GUTTA PERCHA AND HARD CEMENTS

**CONTENTS • Introduction • Pastes • Removal of Pastes • Gutta Percha • Removal of Hard Cements • References**

## INTRODUCTION

This chapter covers the removal of pastes, gutta percha and hard cements from the root canal system. Most of the techniques require the use of magnification and illumination.

## PASTES

The clinician may encounter several pastes that will have been used to obturate the root canal system (Table 4.1).

Historically, some paste systems were advocated for obturating root canals in an attempt to speed up treatment by avoiding the need to adequately disinfect the root canal system. They tend to contain powerful disinfectants to kill bacteria and steroids to reduce inflammation. If left in contact with vital tissue, paraformaldehyde-containing materials or traces of their components can be detected throughout the body.[1] The contents of these pastes are also mutagenic and carcinogenic.[2] Clinical use of materials such as Endomethasone (Specialités-Septodont, Saint Maur-des-Fossés, France) is therefore not accepted in modern endodontic practice.

The modern approach to root canal disinfection by mechanical and chemical means will often require the use of intracanal medicaments. Calcium hydroxide and iodoform-based materials are usually applied to the prepared root canal system as a paste and will need to be removed prior to obturation. Preparations containing mixtures of calcium hydroxide and iodoform, such as Metapex (Technical and

**Table 4.1** *Pastes*

| Material | Radiographic appearance | Appearance | Consistency |
|----------|------------------------|------------|-------------|
| Zinc oxide–eugenol | More radio-opaque than gutta percha | White/grey | Hard. Softer following microleakage |
| Kri paste | White | Yellow | Soft |
| Zinc phosphate | Similar to gutta percha | Creamy yellow/white | Hard. Softer following microleakage |
| Endomethasone | Similar to gutta percha | Grey/brown/pink | Soft |
| Calcium hydroxide | Similar to dentine, depending on content of barium salts | White | Soft |
| Calcium hydroxide/iodoform medicaments | White | Yellow | Soft/spongy |

General Ltd, London, UK), can be slightly more challenging to remove.

## REMOVAL OF PASTES

Pastes normally have a soft consistency, but some materials can become hardened with time. Degradation as a result of bacterial activity will often result in the material becoming sludge-like in consistency.

The majority of soft material can easily be removed during mechanical preparation. Material deeper in the canal and within lateral anatomy can be removed using endosonic irrigation. The vibrating file tip loosens the paste, which is flushed away by irrigant activated by acoustic microstreaming. Sometimes a solvent will also be required (Figure 4.1).

Using a crown-down approach to root canal preparation will allow the bulk of the paste to be removed from the coronal aspect of the root canals early in the preparation sequence. An access cavity should be prepared and refined so that the canal orifices can be identified. An ultrasonic scaler can be used to remove gross deposits of material from the pulp chamber and the superficial parts of the canal orifices. Copious irrigation will help flush away debris (Figures 4.2–4.8).

Following coronal flaring, a pilot channel or glide path is normally prepared to the working length with hand files. This then allows rotary nickel–titanium instruments to be used to rapidly flare the canal to the desired taper. In preparing the canals a significant amount of paste will be removed. Profuse irrigation, perhaps with endosonics and sometimes solvents, will help remove any remaining material.

Solvents include chloroform, Endosolv R and Endosolv E (Specialités-Septodont, Saint Maur-des-Fossés, France). Endosolv R is designed for the removal of phenolic resins, whereas Endosolv E is formulated for the

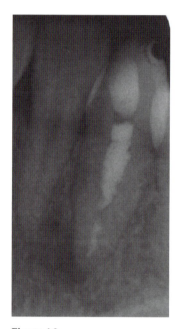

**Figure 4.2**

In this case, a mandibular canine has been obturated using a paste root filling material. There are significant voids between the material and the canal walls. Most of the paste is retained in the coronal part of the root canal, where it will be easiest to remove. The tooth is restorable and there is evidence of periapical periodontitis. Root canal retreatment should offer a good prognosis and will be technically easy to complete. In this case, the access cavity was modified using a long tapered diamond bur to create adequate straight-line access. The paste was then removed with endosonics. The root canal was irrigated using 3% sodium hypochlorite and EDTA and refined with nickel–titanium rotary instruments.

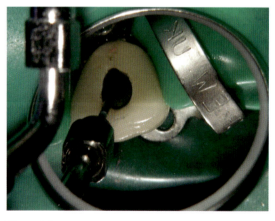

**Figure 4.1**

An endosonic tip can be used to remove paste root fillings. The energized file will help loosen the material and irrigant will wash it away.

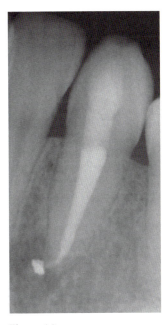

**Figure 4.3**

The case was obturated using a vertically compacted gutta percha technique and the access cavity sealed with resin-modified glass ionomer. In this radiograph, that was taken 6 months following obturation, there has been good evidence of bony healing. A small amount of extruded sealer should not affect the prognosis of treatment.

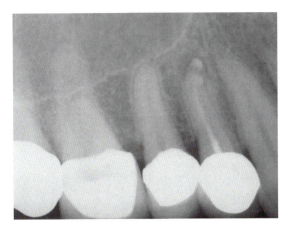

**Figure 4.4**

In this case, a maxillary right first premolar has been obturated using Endomethasone. A small amount of material has been extruded from the apex and careful examination of the radiograph shows that only one canal has been instrumented.

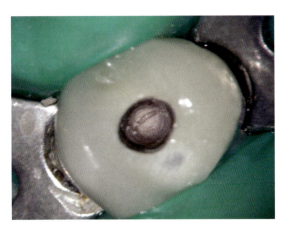

**Figure 4.5**

A view into the access chamber shows Endomethasone paste across the pulp floor. This material was removed using an ultrasonic tip and the pulp space irrigated with 3% sodium hypochlorite.

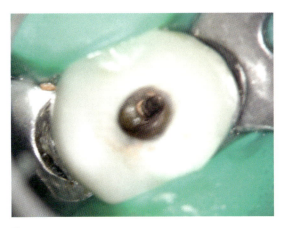

**Figure 4.6**

There is a small amount of retained Endomethasone under the remnants of the roof of the pulp chamber. This was removed very carefully using endosonics and traced across to the unprepared root canal.

removal of eugenol-based cements (Figures 4.9–4.11).[3]

It is notoriously difficult to remove all the material from a root canal system during retreatment. Although the coronal and mid-third may be rendered paste-free relatively easily, apical cleaning and removal from fins, deltas, isthmuses and lateral canals can prove challenging.

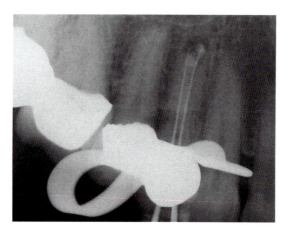

**Figure 4.7**

A diagnostic working length radiograph clearly showing two root canals. Both have been instrumented to their full extent.

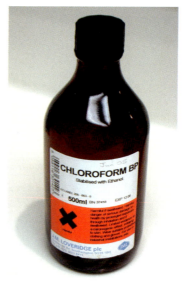

**Figure 4.9**

Chloroform is probably the most effective solvent for gutta percha.

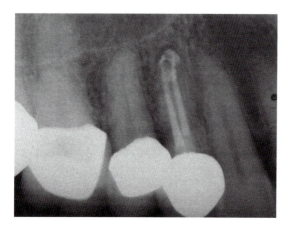

**Figure 4.8**

Following thorough shaping, cleaning and medication with calcium hydroxide, the root canals were obturated with a vertically compacted gutta percha technique. In the apical region there is an isthmus between the two canals.

## Removal of Calcium Hydroxide and Calcium Hydroxide/Iodoform Medicaments

Calcium hydroxide is often used as a root canal medicament. However, there is differing opinion on how successfully the material can be removed prior to obturation. The consensus of opinion suggests that flushing the canal alternately with 17% EDTA and sodium hypochlorite is probably the most effective method.[4,5]

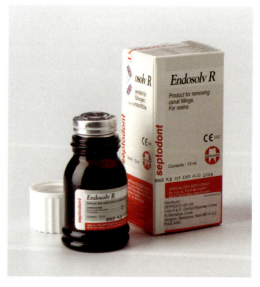

**Figure 4.10**

Endosolve R has been manufactured for the removal of resin-based materials.

Calcium hydroxide/iodoform mixtures such as Metapex are placed into the root canals in a paste form. Although the manufacturer advocates its use as a permanent root canal filling material, it is normally used as a medicament

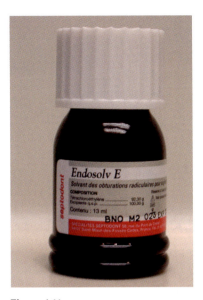

**Figure 4.11**

Endosolve E is useful for the removal of zinc oxide eugenol-based materials.

**Table 4.2** *Removal of pastes*

| Material | Removal |
|----------|---------|
| Zinc oxide–eugenol | Ultrasound and solvents (Endosolv E) |
| Kri paste | Ultrasound |
| Zinc phosphate | Ultrasound |
| Endomethasone | Ultrasound and solvents (Endosolv E) |
| Calcium hydroxide | EDTA and sodium hypochlorite, ultrasound |
| Calcium hydroxide/ iodoform medicaments | Mechanical followed by solvents (chloroform) |

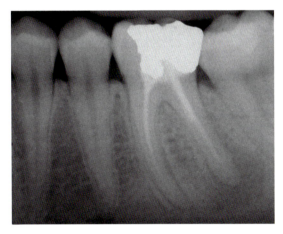

**Figure 4.12**

This mandibular molar has been root treated. However, the root canals are under-prepared and poorly tapered. The root filling material is short of the root canal terminus and poorly condensed. The distal canal contains a post and there is a large periapical radiolucency around the distal root. Such radiolucency can sometimes indicate the presence of a root fracture. While operating in this area, careful examination will be made under high magnification to check that there is not a vertical root fracture. The gutta percha can be easily removed using Gates–Glidden burs and nickel–titanium instruments.

and is removed prior to obturation. The materials become spongy in consistency after a few weeks. The majority of the material will need to be removed mechanically and it can be difficult to achieve this without extrusion. The simplest means is to carefully negotiate the canal with a fine hand file (ISO size 10) to the full working length, making a pilot channel. The final instrument used in preparation is then gently worked to the same length. Modern nickel–titanium instruments are excellent in this respect as the medicament is retrieved and carted coronally when the instrument advances into the canal. Little of the dressing material should be extruded, but any that is will normally be absorbed. A solvent is required to remove the remaining material from within the root canal, and chloroform appears to be effective. This is introduced into the canal in small increments and paper points are used to wick the dissolved material. The process is repeated until the points no longer appear yellow when removed from the canals (Table 4.2, Figures 4.12–4.15).

## GUTTA PERCHA

Gutta percha has been used as a root filling material for over a century.[6] There are many techniques that have been devised for obturation using gutta percha:

- Single cone and sealer.
- Condensed gutta percha techniques:

    Cold lateral condensation
    Warm lateral condensation
    Warm vertical condensation

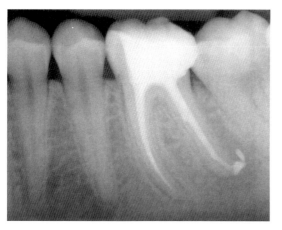

**Figure 4.13**

The case has been thoroughly cleaned and shaped and is now medicated with a calcium hydroxide/iodoform material. The material is radio-opaque and it can be quite useful to take a radiograph to check that the medicament is dispersed effectively throughout the root canal system.

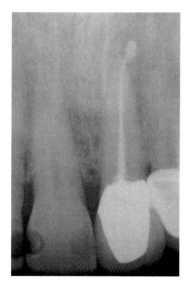

**Figure 4.14**

In this maxillary central incisor, a calcium hydroxide/iodoform-based material has been used as a medicament. Some of the material has been extruded through the apex of the root canal during obturation.

> Thermocompaction
> Hybrid techniques.

- Carrier-based methods.
- Solvent/chloropercha techniques.

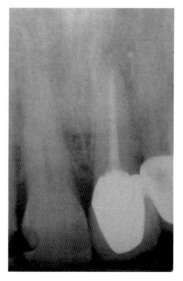

**Figure 4.15**

Three months later the tooth was symptom-free and the buccal sinus tract had healed. Most of the extruded material has been absorbed.

- Cold paste.
- Bonded root filling materials (similar properties to gutta percha but chemically different).

### Single Cone

There will usually be space alongside a single cone root filling that is normally filled with sealer during obturation. The sealer is often degraded by bacterial microleakage, and when a single cone root filling fails this leaves a void.

#### Hedstroem File

Most single cone fillings can be simply removed by engaging the gutta percha with a Hedstroem file carefully wound alongside it. When withdrawn, the file should pull the cone with it (Figures 4.16–4.21).

#### Endosonics

An endosonic file (ISO 15), used with irrigant spray, will break up the sealer layer and aid removal of the cone (Figures 4.22–4.25).

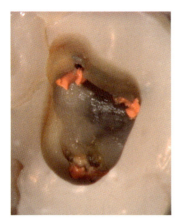

**Figure 4.16**

A single cone root filling in a mandibular molar. Following the preparation of an adequate access cavity, space can be seen alongside the cones of gutta percha. A Hedstroem file can be easily inserted alongside the cone and, when removed, will retrieve the gutta percha. Alternatively, the case could be prepared in the normal manner with nickel–titanium rotary instruments and during coronal flaring the majority of this material will be removed.

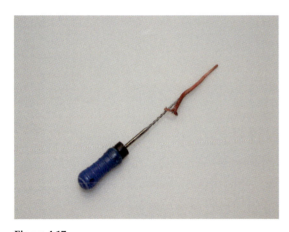

**Figure 4.17**

When engaged, the Hedstroem file will retrieve the gutta percha cone. In this case, the cone is still stuck to the Hedstroem instrument.

## Rotary Nickel–Titanium Instruments

An alternative approach is to tackle the case as if it were an untreated canal, as the root canal will often have been under-prepared and poorly tapered. A crown-down approach is normally used. The coronal aspect is flared first, followed by apical preparation. The cone will undoubtedly be removed during the preparation sequence.

### Over-Extended Gutta Percha

Over-extended gutta percha points can often be retrieved. The canal may be over-filled because the apical part of the root canal has been over-prepared and in many cases zipped. Sometimes, gutta percha is extruded when there has been inflammatory resorption. If the operator fails to achieve an adequate taper or an apical stop during preparation, the gutta percha point can be pushed beyond the apex. In both cases there is often space alongside the cone at the root canal terminus. As much sealer and debris as possible should be removed using irrigants or endosonics on low power before attempting retrieval of the cone. A fine Hedstroem file (ISO 15) is then gently inserted so that it extends 1–2 mm beyond the apical end of the root canal and engages the cone. Gentle pulling should allow the cone to be retrieved. It is important in this instance not to use too large an instrument, as this will result in the extraradicular portion of gutta percha being severed at the apex. Sometimes a braiding technique with two or three Hedstroem files will help dislodge the fragment (Figures 4.26, 4.27).

### Condensed Gutta Percha

The main aim when removing condensed gutta percha is to eliminate as much material from the root canal system by mechanical means before applying solvents. This prevents dissolved gutta percha coating the walls of the access and pulp chamber in a messy smear. Less solvent will also be required.

Even a poor obturating technique can result in material being forced into the complex internal anatomy of the root canal system. For this reason a solvent will always need

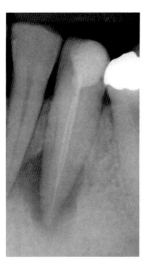

**Figure 4.18**

A single cone root filling in a mandibular canine. The tooth has been under-prepared and poorly root filled. Space can be seen alongside the two cones that have been inserted in the root canals. The coronal restoration was leaking and as a result of persistent infection there is a large periapical radiolucency associated with the tooth. The tooth is restorable, has no periodontal disease associated with it and root canal retreatment should offer a good prognosis. The single cones were easily removed by engaging with a Hedstroem file. The buccal and lingual canals were prepared separately.

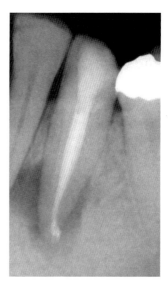

**Figure 4.20**

Following this, the root canal system was obturated with a vertically compacted gutta percha technique and the access cavity filled with a resin-modified glass ionomer.

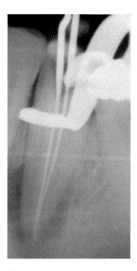

**Figure 4.19**

A diagnostic working length estimation radiograph clearly shows that the canals are patent to their full extent. The case was disinfected using sodium hypochlorite, EDTA and iodine in potassium iodide. Calcium hydroxide was used as a medicament for 1 week.

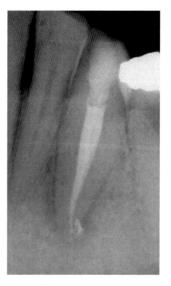

**Figure 4.21**

Six months following obturation, there was good evidence of bony healing.

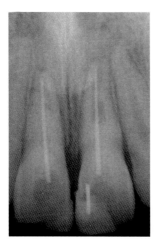

**Figure 4.22**

The single cone root fillings in these immature maxillary central incisors are not sealing the root canals adequately. There is a large area of periapical radio-lucency around both root apices. Because the roots are immature, disinfection should be carried out with the intention of preserving as much root dentine as possible.

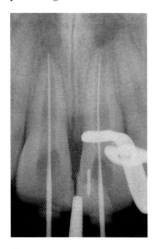

**Figure 4.23**

In this case the single cones were retrieved by irrigating with endosonics. A diagnostic working length estimation radiograph reveals that the root apices are wide and immature. The root canals were cleaned with sodium hypochlorite, EDTA and endosonics. Calcium hydroxide was used as a medicament for 1 week. It is possible to place calcium hydroxide medicament and wait for a barrier to form at the apex. However, if the coronal restoration breaks down, the root canal system can become reinfected. In this case it was decided that MTA would be used to seal the apical portion of the root canal. When working using an operating microscope, it is possible to visualize the apex and mineral trioxide aggregate (MTA) can be packed into this area using gutta percha pluggers.

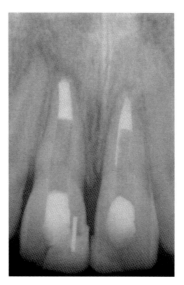

**Figure 4.24**

In this radiograph, mineral trioxide aggregate (MTA) has been placed in the apical region. A damp cotton wool pellet was plugged into the coronal aspect and the access cavity sealed with intermediate restorative material (IRM).

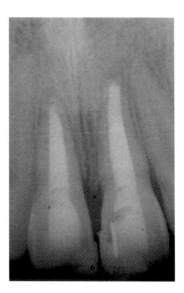

**Figure 4.25**

At a subsequent visit 48 hours later, obturation was completed using thermoplasticized Obtura gutta percha. The access cavities were then sealed with intermediate restorative material (IRM).

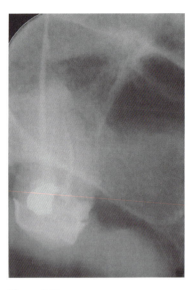

**Figure 4.26**

In this maxillary molar there has been gross over-extension of gutta percha in the palatal canal. There is also a large periapical radiolucency associated with this root. It is likely that the canals were over-instrumented, and infected material was pushed through the apex. In this particular case, the tooth had been left open for some time and was probably highly infected. Retrieval of over-extended gutta percha is dependent on whether the cone has become trapped at the apex. A fine Hedstroem file can sometimes be used to engage the cone and retrieve it.

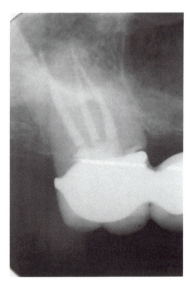

**Figure 4.27**

The gutta percha cone was retrieved and the root canals shaped and disinfected. They were obturated using a vertically compacted gutta percha technique.

to be used when removing condensed gutta percha.[7]

Many ways of removing the bulk of gutta percha have been suggested, including Gates–Glidden burs, rotary instruments, heat and lasers (Figures 4.28–4.30).[8–13]

### Gates–Glidden Burs

A Gates–Glidden bur size 2 or 3 is a very efficient instrument for penetrating and removing gutta percha from the coronal part of the root canal. The bur, which is rotated at 2000–3000 rpm, thermoplasticizes and removes gutta percha simultaneously (Figure 4.31).

### *Heat*

Heat can be used to remove the bulk of gutta percha from the coronal part of the root canal. A heated instrument, or electrically heated pluggers such as the Touch and Heat or System B (SybronEndo, Orange, CA, USA), are useful. Place the plugger in the canal hot and allow to cool slightly. Small amounts

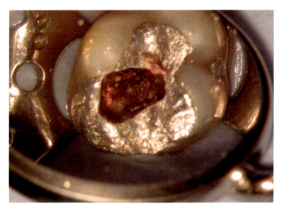

**Figure 4.28**

In this case, a tooth has been root filled using a gutta percha technique. However, on preparing an access cavity it was apparent that the roof of the pulp chamber had not been removed. Root canal treatment had been carried out through the pulp horns.

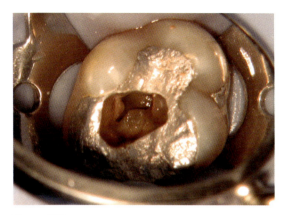

**Figure 4.29**

Cleaning the access with sodium hypochlorite revealed the roof of the pulp chamber. The access cavity had to be refined to provide straight-line access to the orifices of the root canals.

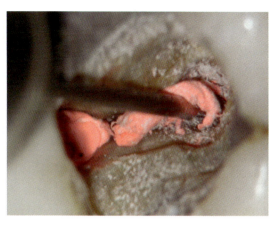

**Figure 4.31**

A Gates–Glidden bur is a very efficient means of removing gutta percha from the coronal aspect of the root canals.

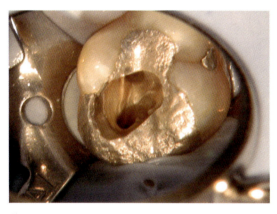

**Figure 4.30**

The access was refined using a non-end-cutting tungsten carbide bur. The coronal aspect of the root canals was prepared with nickel–titanium rotary instruments. A trough was created from the mesiobuccal canal in the direction of the palatal canal to ascertain whether there was a second mesiobuccal canal.

of gutta percha will be removed with the plugger.

## Nickel–Titanium Rotary Instruments

Rotary nickel–titanium instruments such as ProFiles (Denstply-Maillefer, Ballaigues,

Switzerland) offer an efficient means of removing gutta percha and can be used further apically than Gates–Glidden burs.[7,12,14] If the canal has previously been well prepared, a rotary instrument should be selected that has a smaller taper than that of the prepared canal to avoid binding and potential separation. In other words, the instrument is working mainly within the mass of gutta percha. If the canal has been under-prepared, then mechanical preparation is completed in the normal fashion but a solvent can be applied to help aid removal of the gutta percha (Figures 4.32, 4.33).

## Specialized Instruments

There are specific gutta percha removal instruments available, such as the GPX (Brasseler USA, Savannah, GA, USA). This instrument is rotated in a speed-reducing handpiece and has cutting flutes arranged in a reverse screw thread. Gutta percha is thermoplasticized and withdrawn from the canal by the action of the flutes. There is a risk of fracture if excessive force is applied, when the instrument is rotated too quickly, or is made to work around curvatures in the root canal.

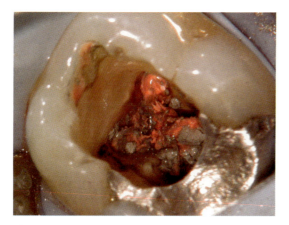

**Figure 4.32**

In this retreatment case the root canals have been obturated with condensed gutta percha. The filling material from a previous attempt has been removed from the access cavity, which is oversized. This provided good visibility of the pulp floor.

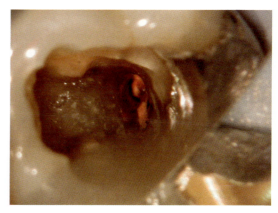

**Figure 4.34**

Following mechanical removal, there were small tags of gutta percha remaining in the root canal. These were visualized using the operating microscope and retrieved with a Hedstroem file and micro-debrider.

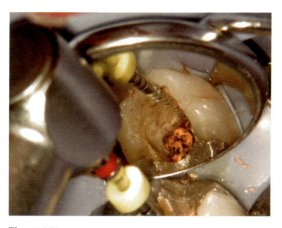

**Figure 4.33**

The condensed gutta percha was retrieved in this case using a Profile instrument. This was rotated at approximately 350 rpm to machine and withdraw gutta percha from the root canals.

Following the use of mechanical instruments, any small tags that remain can be visualized under the operating microscope with good illumination and magnification. They are then retrieved with a Hedstroem file or micro-debrider (Maillefer, Ballaigues, Switzerland). It is sometimes useful to run an instrument along the lateral borders of the

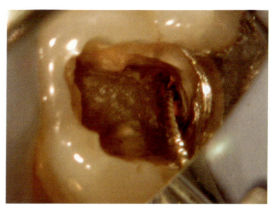

**Figure 4.35**

A Hedstroem file being used to retrieve small tags of remaining gutta percha.

canal, especially if it is ribbon-shaped, to remove any gross deposits of material that have been compacted into lateral grooves and fins (Figures 4.34–4.37).

Solvents

Any remaining gutta percha can be removed using a solvent and these include:

- chloroform BP (stabilized in ethanol)
- eucalyptus oil

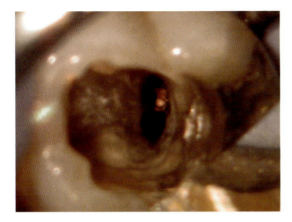

**Figure 4.36**

Tiny fragments remaining at the apex were dissolved with chloroform and absorbed onto paper points.

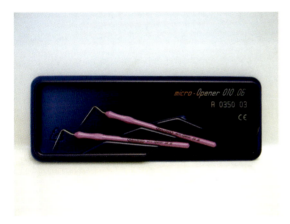

**Figure 4.37**

Micro-openers are useful for retrieving small items from the root canals when using the operating microscope. They can also be used to find the orifices of root canals.

- rectified turpentine
- xylene
- methyl chloroform
- halothane.

Solvents can usually be obtained from larger pharmacies or chemical companies and they vary in their effectiveness.[15] Chloroform is highly effective and probably the most popular solvent for endodontic use. Some concern has been expressed about the cytotoxic effects

of gutta percha solvents.[16] However, it is unlikely that with careful use the small amounts of chloroform required in endodontic retreatment would be hazardous.

Chloroform is introduced a few drops at a time to the root canals. It should be drawn up in a glass or polypropylene syringe. Normally, less than 1 ml will be required for a retreatment case. The rubber dam will dissolve should the solvent come into contact with it.

Initially, a Hedstroem file can be used to remove dissolved material. The file is wiped clean on a gauze between insertions. Following this, more solvent is placed into the canal and paper point used to wick the dissolved material from lateral canals and fins. When the paper points are no longer coloured on removal, the root canals should be free of gutta percha (Figures 4.38–4.46).

### Carrier-Based Gutta Percha

#### Thermafil

There have been several carrier-based obturating devices marketed for use in endodontics. Most consist of a metal or plastic carrier covered in alpha-phase gutta percha. Thermafil (Dentsply-Maillefer, Ballaigues, Switzerland) is probably one of the most well known.

Early Thermafil carriers were made of titanium but were soon replaced by a plastic alternative. The most recent development is a V-shaped cross section on the 0.04 tapered plastic carrier that is aimed at making retreatment simpler. The removal of Thermafil is not considered to be a major problem in retreatment.[17–20] Removing the carrier is important in speeding up the process and allowing removal of the gutta percha (Figure 4.47).[21]

#### Hedstroem Files

Using magnification and illumination, it is possible to uncover the carrier and insert a Hedstroem file alongside by gently screwing it clockwise. Occasionally, the carrier can be removed by withdrawing the file by hand. If more force is required, the file can be clamped in a pair of artery forceps and

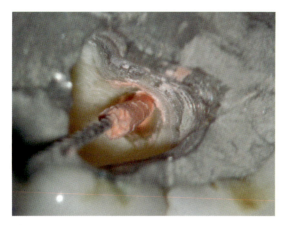

**Figure 4.38**

Following retrieval of the majority of gutta percha from the root canals, a solvent is used to dissolve the remaining material. In this case, chloroform has been introduced to the root canals and a Hedstroem file used to retrieve the mass of dissolved gutta percha. To start with, a large amount of gutta percha can be seen coating the Hedstroem file. This is cleaned on a gauze before reinsertion.

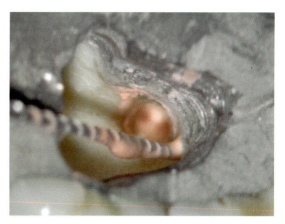

**Figure 4.40**

After a third application of chloroform, there was little gutta percha being retrieved on the Hedstroem file and wicking was started with paper points.

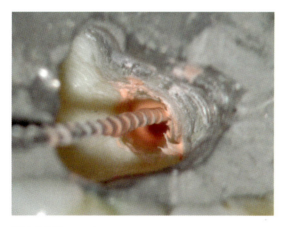

**Figure 4.39**

After a while, the amount of gutta percha coating the Hedstroem file will be reduced. Additional increments of chloroform will be required to dissolve the remaining gutta percha as it evaporates.

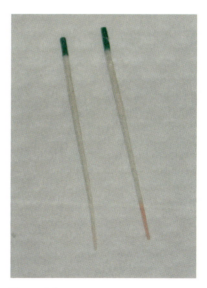

**Figure 4.41**

Wicking is carried out until the paper points are not discoloured when retrieved from the root canals. On the right-hand side, the cone is stained slightly pink from dissolved gutta percha, whereas on the left, the cone is virtually unchanged. In this case the root canal system should be devoid of gutta percha.

leverage applied by rotating about a cotton wool roll placed on the adjacent tooth. The remaining gutta percha can be removed in a similar manner to well-condensed gutta percha (Figures 4.48, 4.49).

When Thermafil has been in place for a number of years, the gutta percha can become quite hard. In this instance, it is difficult to make progress with the Hedstroem file. A well

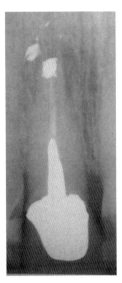

**Figure 4.42**

In this case a maxillary central incisor has been restored with a post core and crown. It has already been root filled and apisected using an amalgam retrograde technique. There is a periapical radiolucency associated with the tooth. In this instance root canal retreatment should be carried out first. The gutta percha can easily be removed with Gates–Glidden burs and the amalgam root end filling visualized with the operating microscope. The root canal space is then cleaned with sodium hypochlorite and endosonics.

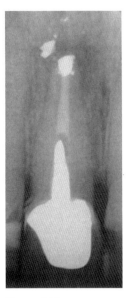

**Figure 4.43**

Due to the shortened root length and requirement for a post, it could be difficult to achieve sufficient length of gutta percha to produce an adequate seal (minimum 4 mm). Therefore, in this case, the root canal was obturated with mineral trioxide aggregate (MTA).

can be created in the orifice of the canal using a size 3 or 4 Gates–Glidden bur, into which solvent such as chloroform is placed. The gutta percha will soften sufficiently to enable a Hedstroem file to be introduced alongside the carrier.

## Nickel–Titanium Rotary Instruments

The plastic carrier can sometimes be removed using a rotary nickel–titanium instrument 0.04 taper, rotated at 600–1200 rpm. The file should be rotated in the groove of the carrier and advanced with light pressure. Frictional heat will melt the gutta percha, allowing the instrument to advance apically and create a pilot channel. Once resistance is felt, a 0.06 taper instrument is used at normal working speed of 300 rpm to grip the carrier and extract it.

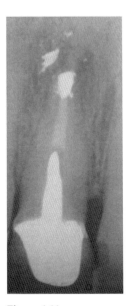

**Figure 4.44**

Six months following obturation, there were good signs of early bony healing.

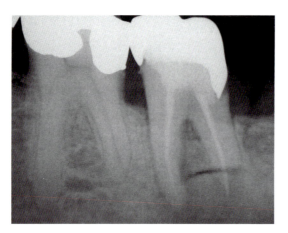

**Figure 4.45**

In this mandibular molar, the root canals were under-prepared and the root filling was inadequate. In the distal canal there may have been some resorption, leading to over-extension of gutta percha or perhaps the gutta percha was over-extended during obturation. There is a minor periodontal defect on the mesial aspect of the tooth, but it is restorable. Root canal retreatment should offer a good prognosis. The existing root filling was removed using a combination of Gates–Glidden burs and nickel–titanium rotary instruments. It was then disinfected with 4% sodium hypochlorite and EDTA. Calcium hydroxide was used as a medicament between appointments.

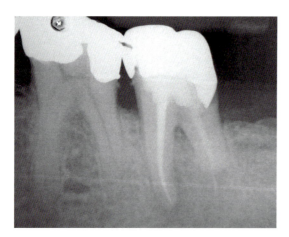

**Figure 4.46**

Due to the short root length in the distal canal and the large diameter of the apical terminus, it was decided that mineral trioxide aggregate (MTA) would be used as the obturating material. Six months following obturation, there is good evidence of bony healing. It was not possible to remove all the over-extended gutta percha and some of this has been retained beyond the apex of the distal root. The coronal restoration will now require replacement.

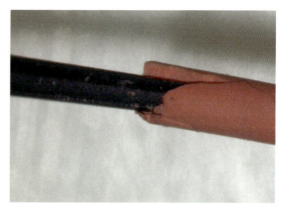

**Figure 4.47**

A small amount of gutta percha has been removed from a Thermafil obturator to reveal the V-shaped groove. It is into this groove that the Hedstroem file can be inserted to remove the Thermafil carrier from the root canals.

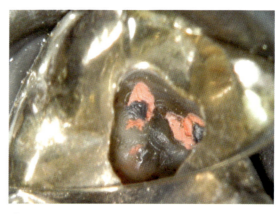

**Figure 4.48**

In this mandibular molar, the root canals have been obturated using Thermafil. An access cavity has been prepared and the black carriers can be easily distinguished from the gutta percha. Space is made alongside them to aid retrieval.

If the carrier seems resistant, a Hedstroem file and solvent can be used. The remaining gutta percha can be removed in a similar manner to well-condensed gutta percha.

### Quickfill

This system utilized nickel–titanium carriers covered in gutta percha to obturate the root

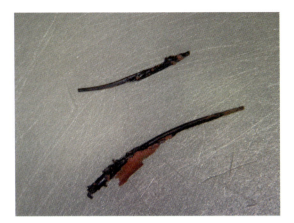

**Figure 4.49**

In this case, the cones in the mesial canals were retrieved using the Hedstroem files. The area where the Hedstroem file engaged the cone can be seen.

canal system. Removal is relatively simple when the heads of the carriers have been retained. First, gutta percha around the head of the carrier is removed with a Gates–Glidden bur. The carrier is then removed using Stieglitz forceps. The remaining gutta percha can be removed in a similar manner to well-condensed gutta percha.

If the carrier has been severed below orifice level, then it will have to be uncovered using Gates–Glidden burs or solvents under magnification and illumination. It can usually be removed using either the instrument removal system (IRS) or braiding (see fractured instruments) (Figures 4.50, 4.51).

## Other Systems

### Solvent/Chloropercha

Canals obturated using gutta percha and solvent techniques can be treated in a similar manner to condensed gutta percha.

### Gutta Flow

Gutta Flow (Coltene Whaledent Ltd, Sussex, UK) is a cold gutta percha filling system that utilizes a silicone matrix and shredded gutta percha. It can be removed using similar techniques to condensed gutta percha.

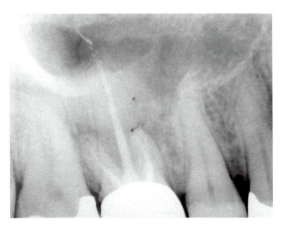

**Figure 4.50**

This molar has been obturated using Quickfill. The carrier in this case is made of nickel–titanium and can be removed in a similar way to separated instruments. The carrier is coated in gutta percha and normally it is easier to remove some of the material first before attempting retrieval of the carrier.

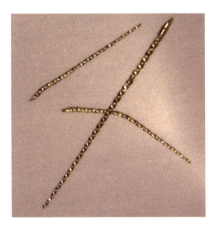

**Figure 4.51**

The Quickfill carriers were all retrieved using endosonics, Hedstroem files and Stieglitz forceps.

### Resilon

Resilon (Resilon Research LLC, Madison, CT, USA) is a thermoplastic, synthetic, polymer-based root canal filling material. The material contains bioactive glass and radio-opaque fillers. It performs like gutta percha and has similar handling properties. For retreatment purposes, it may be softened with heat, or dissolved with solvents such as chloroform. Epiphany (Pentron Clinical Technologies, LLC, Wallingford, CT, USA) is a dual curable dental resin composite sealer that is used with Resilon. It is claimed that the resin can impregnate dentinal tubules,[22] providing a bond between the mass of obturating material and the wall of the root canal. In a retreatment situation, this hybrid layer may need to be removed mechanically by enlarging the canal (Figure 4.52).

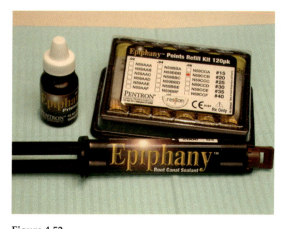

**Figure 4.52**

Epiphany is a bondable root filling material and can be removed in a similar manner to conventional gutta percha.

## REMOVAL OF HARD CEMENTS

There are several hard cements that could be encountered during root canal retreatment (Table 4.3).

Hard materials are one of the most challenging to remove from the root canal system, as there is an increased risk of damaging the tooth.[23] Set cement will probably have to be removed by mechanical means using burs or ultrasonic tips.[24] Sometimes a solvent may be available if the material can be identified (Figures 4.53, 4.54).

When the root filling has been poorly placed or microbial leakage has undermined a material, there may be voids created along the canal wall interface that will allow the introduction of instruments and consequently aid removal.

Good illumination and magnification, preferably with a microscope, will allow the operator to distinguish between the filling material and the root canal wall. This should reduce the risk of perforation.

Tungsten carbide burs (D 0205 LN burs, Dentsply-Maillefer, Ballaigues, Switzerland) can be used to remove material from the most coronal part of the root canal. Diamond-coated ultrasonic tips used in a Piezon-type ultrasonic machine are particularly useful. These can be used with or without waterspray but, when used dry, the assistant will need to

**Table 4.3** *Cements*

| Material | Radiographic appearance | Appearance | Consistency |
| --- | --- | --- | --- |
| SPAD (Bakelite) | More radio-opaque than gutta percha | White/grey | Hard |
| AH26 (resin) | More radio-opaque than gutta percha | Creamy yellow/white | Hard |
| Zinc phosphate | Similar to gutta percha | Creamy yellow/white | Hard. Softer following microleakage |
| Resorcinol–formalin | Similar to gutta percha | Red/pink may stain tooth substance | Very hard, glassy |
| Glass ionomer | Similar to gutta percha | Creamy yellow/white | Hard |
| N2 (zinc oxide–eugenol) | More radio-opaque than gutta percha | Creamy yellow/white | Hard |

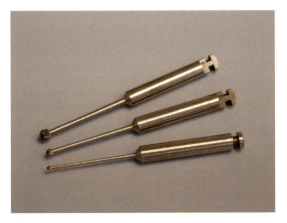

**Figure 4.53**

Swan-necked tungsten carbide LN burs are an invaluable tool for removing cements from the root canal. They should always be used with direct vision, preferably with an operating microscope to prevent the risk of perforation.

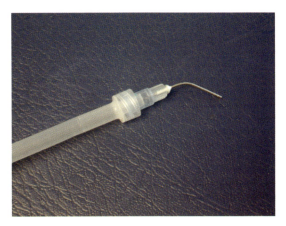

**Figure 4.55**

A disposable Stropko-style irrigator with an Endo-Eze tip fitted. The assistant can puff air across the operating site to disperse dentine chips as they are created by the ultrasonic tip.

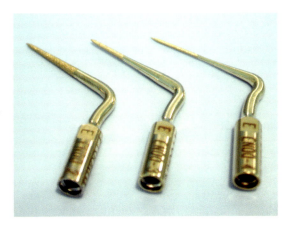

**Figure 4.54**

The Pro-Ultra endosonic tips. These tips are all diamond coated and can be used to retrieve cements from the coronal to mid-third of the root canal.

**Table 4.4** *Removal of cements*

| Material | Removal |
|----------|---------|
| SPAD (Bakelite) | Ultrasound, may be difficult |
| AH26 (resin) | Ultrasound |
| Zinc phosphate | Ultrasound |
| Resorcinol–formalin | Ultrasound, solvents (Endosolv R) |
| Glass ionomer | Ultrasound |
| N2 (zinc oxide–eugenol) | Ultrasound, solvents (Endosolv E) |

puff air from a 3:1 syringe onto the field to clear dust particles for aspiration. Occasionally, chips may prevent a clear view of the interface between material and root wall. In this instance irrigation with EDTA for 2 minutes followed by air drying will usually clear the microscopic field. The Stropko irrigator (Obtura Corporation, Fenton, MO, USA) is a useful addition to the armamentarium when working with a microscope and allows easy drying of the operating field when working at higher magnifications (Figure 4.55).

Solvents for set cements are notoriously slow-acting, and removal using this method can be extremely laborious and time-consuming.[25] Solvent is applied to the material and allowed to react. An endodontic instrument is used to remove any softened material. The solvent is replenished and the process repeated. Endosolv R is designed for the removal of phenolic resins, whereas Endosolv E is formulated for the removal of eugenol-based cements. Chloroform may also be useful for some types of set cement. Resorcinol–formalin-based materials are notoriously difficult to remove, and even solvents may prove inefficient. The manufacturers of Endosolv R recommend that the solvent is sealed into the root canal orifice for several days, during which the cement should soften.[26] Dimethyl sulfoxide (DMSO, Sigma-Aldrich, San Diego, CA, USA) has been suggested for removal of this material (Table 4.4).[25]

## REFERENCES

1. Block RM, Lewis RD, Hirsh J, Coffey J, Langeland K. Systemic distribution of [$^{14}$C] labelled paraformaldehhyde incorporated within formocresol following pulpotomies in dogs. *Journal of Endodontics*, 1983; **9**: 176–189.

2. Ørstavik D, Hongslo JK. Mutagenicity of endodontic sealers. *Biomaterials* 1985; **6**: 129–132.

3. Vranas RN, Hartwell GR, Moon PC. The effect of endodontic solutions on resorcinol-formalin paste. *Journal of Endodontics* 2003; **29**: 69–72.

4. Lambriandis T, Margeloo J, Beltes P. Removal efficiency of calcium hydroxide dressing from the root canals. *Journal of Endodontics* 1999; **25**: 85–88.

5. Calt S, Serper A. Dentinal tubule penetration of root canal sealers after root canal dressing with calcium hydroxide. *Journal of Endodontics* 1999; **25**: 431–433.

6. Bowman GA. Root filling. *Missouri Dental Journal* 1876; **8**: 372–376.

7. Ferreira JJ, Rhodes JS, Pitt Ford TR. The efficacy of gutta-percha removal using ProFiles. *International Endodontic Journal* 2001; **34**: 267–274.

8. Hülsmann M, Stotz S. Efficacy, cleaning ability and safety of different devices for gutta-percha removal in root canal retreatment. *International Endodontic Journal* 1997; **30**: 227–233.

9. Bramante CM, Betti LV. Efficacy of Quantec rotary instruments for gutta-percha removal. *International Endodontic Journal* 2000; **33**: 463–467.

10. Betti LV, Bramanate CM. Quantec SC rotary instruments versus hand files for gutta percha removal in root canal retreatment. *International Endodontic Journal* 2001; **34**: 514–519.

11. Viducic D, Jukic S, Karlovic Z, Bozic Z, Miletic I, Anic I. Removal of gutta percha from root canals using Nd:YAG laser. *International Endodontic Journal* 2003; **36**: 670–673.

12. Hülsmann M, Bluhm V. Efficacy, cleaning ability and safety of different rotary NiTi instruments in root canal retreatment. *International Endodontic Journal* 2004; **37**: 468–476.

13. Masiero AV, Barletta FB. Effectiveness of different techniques for removing gutta percha during retreatment. *International Endodontic Journal* 2005; **38**: 2–7.

14. Baratto Filho F, Ferreira EL, Fariniuk LF. Efficiency of the 0.04 taper ProFile during the re-treatment of gutta-percha-filled root canals. *International Endodontic Journal* 2002; **35**: 651–654.

15. Wennberg A, Ørstavik D. Evaluation of alternatives to chloroform in endodontic practice. *Endodontics and Dental Traumatology* 1989; **5**: 234–237.

16. Barbosa SV, Burkard DH, Spångberg LSW. Cytotoxic effects of gutta percha solvents. *Journal of Endodontics* 1994; **20**: 6–8.

17. Bertrand MF, Pellegrino JC, Rocca JP, Klinghofer A, Bolla M. Removal of Thermafil root canal filling material. *Journal of Endodontics* 1997; **23**: 54–57.

18. Frajlich SR, Goldberg F, Massone EJ, Cantarini C, Artaza LP. Comparative study of retreatment of Thermafil and lateral condensation endodontic fillings. *International Endodontic Journal* 1998; **31**: 354–357.

19. Wolcott JF, Himel VT, Hicks ML. Thermafil retreatment using a new 'System B' technique or a solvent. *Journal of Endodontics* 1999; **25**: 761–764.

20. Ibarrola JL, Knowles KI, Ludlow MO. Retrievability of Thermafil plastic cores using organic solvents. *Journal of Endodontics* 1993; **19**: 417–418.

21. Wilcox LR. Thermafil retreatment with and without chloroform solvent. *Journal of Endodontics* 1993; **19**: 563–566.

22. Shipper G, Ørstavik D, Teixeira FB, Trope M. An evaluation of microbial leakage in roots filled with a thermoplastic

synthetic polymer-based root canal filling material (Resilon). *Journal of Endodontics* 2004; **30**: 342–347.

23. Jeng HW, El Deeb. Removal of hard paste fillings from the root canal by ultrasonic instrumentation. *Journal of Endodontics* 1997; **13**: 295–298.

24. Friedman S, Stabholz A, Tamse A. Endodontic retreatment – case selection and technique. *Journal of Endodontics* 1990; **16**: 543–549.

25. Gambrel MG, Hartwell G, Moon PC, Cardon JW. The effect of endodontic solutions on resorcinol-formalin paste in teeth. *Journal of Endodontics* 2005; **31**: 25–29.

26. Endosolv. Product for removing canal fillings. Manufacturers insert. Septodont, St Maur-des-Fosses, France; 2000.

# 5 REMOVAL OF SILVER POINTS AND SEPARATED INSTRUMENTS

CONTENTS • Introduction • The Microscope • Removal of Silver Points • Removing Separated Instruments • Removal of Nickel–Titanium Instruments • References

## INTRODUCTION

The use of operating microscopes in endodontics has seen the possibilities for endodontic treatment and retreatment expand dramatically.[1] Retrieval of objects from within the root canal system to allow adequate disinfection can now be achieved where it was once impossible. An operating microscope is an invaluable tool in endodontics and one most endodontists would consider essential for carrying out the techniques described in this chapter. The published success rates for removal of fractured instruments from root canals using modern techniques have ranged from 68 to 87%.[2–4] The majority of instruments requiring removal would appear to be rotary and most seem to fail in curved root canals. Decreased success was seen when the removal time was in excess of 45–60 minutes, the fragment was positioned apically and ultrasound was used for longer.[4]

## THE MICROSCOPE

Most practitioners have had experience of using loupes, and these can provide magnification in the range ×2 to ×6. Direct illumination is invaluable and can be provided by a headlamp that is attached to the glasses. As magnifications become higher, loupes tend to be heavier and more unwieldy and the field of view is decreased. This means that small movements by the operator or by the patient can result in loss of view of the operating field.

Since the operating microscope is essentially fixed, this problem is much easier to manage and consequently higher magnifications can be provided and successfully used while operating (Figure 5.1).

Microscopes can provide magnifications in the range ×3 to ×30. Low magnifications are excellent for general work and have a wider field of view and good depth of focus. Higher magnifications are used for specific tasks such as hunting for missed canals and retrieving separated instruments. The field of view and depth

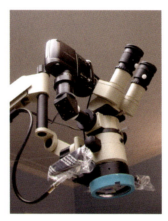

**Figure 5.1**

The operating microscope is invaluable in endodontics for treatment, retreatment and surgical procedures. This global microscope has three steps of magnification. It has a beam splitter, which allows the mounting of a digital camera. The camera can be used to take still photos or to provide a continuous video stream for viewing on a computer screen. Cross-infection barriers are placed on the handles and over the main lens; they are changed between patients.

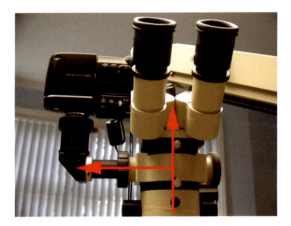

**Figure 5.2**

The beam splitter divides the light (red arrows) from the objective and diverts it into the eyepieces and other accessory devices: these include additional assistant viewing binoculars, a mini camera or digital camera.

of focus will be reduced and, for these reasons, it can be easier to use the lower magnifications when taking photographs for records.

The overall magnification is determined by the eyepiece, focal length of the binoculars, the selected magnification lens and the objective lens. Eyepieces normally have magnifications in the range ×6.6 to ×20. They have rubber cups at the end, which are turned down when the operator is wearing glasses. The eyepieces are arranged as binoculars. It is sometimes useful to have inclinable binoculars, especially if different operators are using the same microscope.

In order to use the microscope, the operator must first carry out parfocalling. On high magnification each eye is focused independently on an object using the eyepiece adjustment. Illumination is normally provided by fibre optic cable from a quartz halogen, xenon or metal halide light source. A halogen light can give a yellowish tinge, whereas xenon is similar to bright sunlight. In order to mount a camera on the microscope, a beam splitter will be required to direct the image in two directions (Figure 5.2).

## REMOVAL OF SILVER POINTS

Silver points are no longer considered an appropriate method of obturating root canals.

They were first introduced into endodontics in 1933. A silver cone that corresponded to the final preparation size was cemented in the root canal with a sealer or zinc phosphate cement. Tags of the coronal ends were retained in the pulp chamber and embedded in zinc oxide–eugenol or zinc phosphate.[5,6] Retention of these tags will make removal easier. Points that have sheared off at the level of the pulp floor or sub-orifice regions and those that are well cemented can be much more challenging to retrieve.

Many silver point root treatments have been carried out and the technique has been widely used on a global scale. Unfortunately, many have subsequently failed. The silver point technique could be abused and completed from a technical perspective without following fundamental biological principles that are now accepted in modern endodontics. Even when canals are under-prepared, a stiff silver cone can be forced to the full working length without proper cleaning. Radiographically, the operator may be content that the seal is adequate but biologically the case could be failing. A poor seal would be produced by the cement and rigid cone and when recolonization of the root canal occurs through coronal microleakage, the root canal filling fails and the cones corrode (Figures 5.3–5.9).[7–10]

Despite the technique no longer being considered suitable for obturating root canals, it still appears to be in use today. There are numerous techniques that have been described to remove silver cones;[10–13] the ease with which this can be achieved will depend upon the amount of retained point in the pulp chamber and the degree of microleakage that has occurred, causing dissolution of the cement.

## Removal of Poorly Cemented Silver Points

When there has been significant microleakage, the cement lute will often have been degraded and the silver point may even be loose in the root canal. If a tag has been left in the pulp chamber, retrieval should be relatively easy. It is important when removing core material to avoid cutting through the

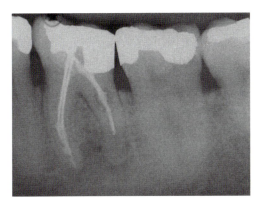

**Figure 5.3**

This mandibular first molar has been root filled using a silver point root filling technique. The root canals have been inadequately prepared and there has been significant microleakage. Paste can be seen both in the coronal aspect of the distal root canal and in the apical third of the mesial canals. There is a large periapical area that extends around both root tips and an area of internal resorption in the distal root. The tooth is restorable and there are no significant periodontal problems surrounding it. Root canal retreatment is therefore justified and should have good prognosis.

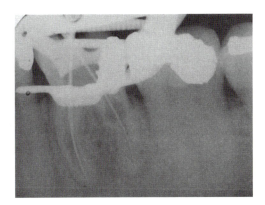

**Figure 5.4**

Following refinement of the access cavity, the root canals were thoroughly irrigated using sodium hypochlorite. A diagnostic working length estimation radiograph revealed that the canals in this tooth were completely patent. Some refinement in the preparation was required using tapered nickel–titanium rotary instruments. The root canal space was then disinfected with 3% sodium hypochlorite and EDTA.

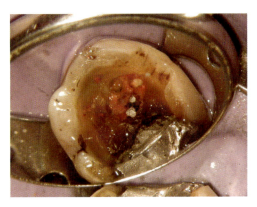

**Figure 5.5**

When there has been significant microleakage, the silver points are generally much easier to remove. In this case, removal of the temporary restoration from the existing access cavity revealed that the pulp roof had not been adequately removed. The small hole that had been created was filled with Endomethasone paste and the heads of the silver points were visible within this. The Endomethasone was removed using endosonic tips and CPR 5, following which the silver points could be removed very simply using Hedstroem files and Stieglitz forceps. The roof of the pulp chamber was then removed with a non-end-cutting tungsten carbide bur to provide visualization of the pulp floor.

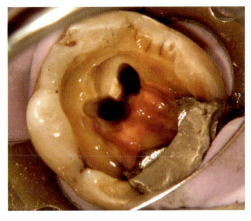

**Figure 5.6**

The mesial canals following coronal flaring and refinement of the access chamber. The pulp floor was stained pink by the Endomethasone paste that had previously been used as a root filling material.

tags. Under microscopic magnification and illumination, the core material is best removed using an ultrasonic tip such as the CT4, CPR 2 or 3, BUC-1 or 3, or Pro-Ultra

Endo tip 2 with or without irrigant spray. Ultrasonic energy will cause the core material to fragment but leave the tags of silver cone intact. It is very tempting to try to remove the core material using a bur but this will undoubtedly result in severing the cone, making retrieval more difficult.

Once the core material has been removed, the access cavity is thoroughly irrigated with sodium hypochlorite or iodine solution.

Cement around the coronal orifices of the silver cones can be removed very carefully using an endosonic tip (ISO size 15 file) on low power together with irrigant. If the point is loose, it can be gripped with Stieglitz forceps and withdrawn (Figure 5.10).

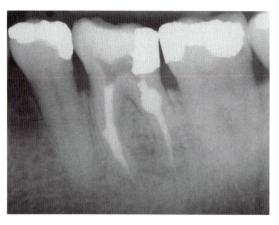

**Figure 5.7**

Obturation completed using a vertically compacted gutta technique and Obtura thermoplasticized gutta percha. A foam sponge has been placed in the pulp chamber and the access sealed with intermediate restorative material (IRM). This tooth was due to be restored within 2 weeks of completion of the root canal treatment.

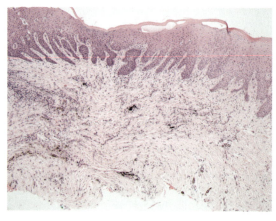

**Figure 5.9**

A biopsy of the sinus tract was taken and a histopathology report requested. Under low magnification, silver particles can clearly be seen dispersed through the epithelium.

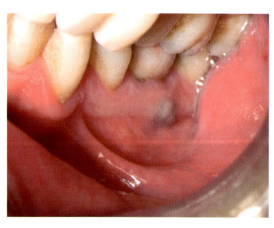

**Figure 5.8**

The clinical view of the mandibular molar showing a sinus tract on the buccal mucosa. This healed following initial cleaning, shaping and medication with calcium hydroxide. The area was stained black. This was a result of corrosion of the silver points in the root canal.

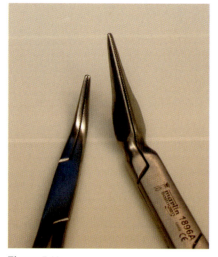

**Figure 5.10**

Retrieval of objects from the access chamber can be achieved using forceps. The Stieglitz forceps are modified to make the beaks slimmer. Micro artery forceps can also be useful.

Alternatively, a Hedstroem file can be carefully inserted alongside the point by screwing it gently in a clockwise direction and, when engaged, can be withdrawn together with the point (Figures 5.11–5.16).

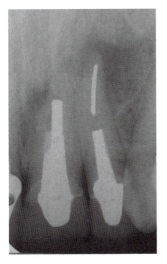

**Figure 5.11**

These maxillary incisors have been restored using cast post cores and crowns. The lateral incisor has a silver point root filling in the apical third. The root canal is undoubtedly infected as there is a large area of periapical radiolucency surrounding it. Root canal retreatment in this instance will offer the best opportunity of cleaning the infected root canal.

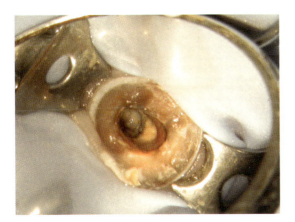

**Figure 5.12**

Following removal of the post using ultrasonics, the operating microscope can be used to view down the root canal. At this stage there is some cement retained on the root canal wall. This can easily be removed with an ultrasonic tip such as the CPR 5.

## The Meitrac (Hager & Meisinger, Neuss, Germany)

This system consists of trephines and extractors that are designed to remove intraradicular obstructions of different diameters. The Meitrac I System is designed for broken instruments with diameters of 0.15–0.5 mm. The Meitrac II System is designed for the retrieval of silver points of diameters 0.5–0.9 mm. The trephine drill is effectively a hollow cylinder and can be used to mill cement or dentine away from around the point at orifice level.

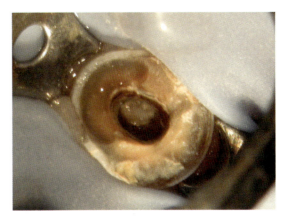

**Figure 5.13**

The canal was then irrigated with sodium hypochlorite.

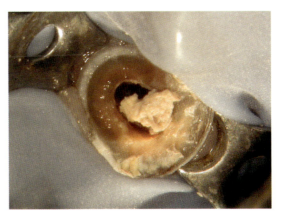

**Figure 5.14**

A piece of cotton wool had been retained in the root canal. This had been present for over 20 years!

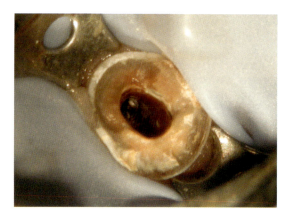

**Figure 5.15**

Having removed the cotton wool and irrigated the root canal thoroughly using sodium hypochlorite and EDTA, the head of the apical silver point was clearly visible. It was now possible to insert a Hedstroem file alongside the point. Endosonics were also used. The point was relatively loose and could easily be retrieved.

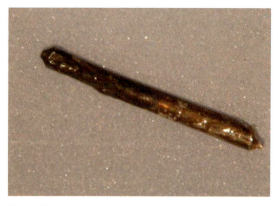

**Figure 5.16**

The silver point shows corrosion products on its tip. The coronal end is intact and clearly shows where it was severed during an apical silver point technique.

The remover consists of two hollow tubes that fit inside one another. The internal tube has slim jaws that grip the point as the handles are depressed. The Meitrac system may be useful for removing silver points in the coronal part of the root canal. However, the trephine drill and removers are too large for use below orifice level (Figure 5.17).

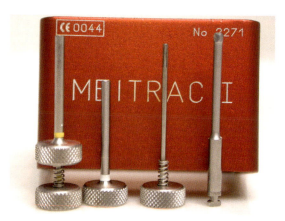

**Figure 5.17**

The Meitrac II system for removal of small objects.

## Cancellier and Needles

The Cancellier kit (Maillefer, Ballaigues, Switzerland) consists of a series of graded hollow tubes that are held in a long handle. Tubes are matched to the size of point that is to be removed. Cyanoacrylate cement (superglue) is then used to bond the point and tube together before removal.[14] Methacrylate monomer can be used to speed up the setting of the glue. The amount of overlap (in the range of 1–3 mm) and snugness of fit have been shown to be significant factors to obtaining good adhesion. The adhesive requires a setting time of 5 minutes for maximum bonding, except when there is loose fit between the extractor and the silver point.[15] An alternative method is to use hypodermic needles[16] or an appropriate Endo-Eze tip (Ultradent Products Inc, South Jordan, USA). There is no risk of bonding the tube to the tooth with cyanoacrylate, but the degree of adhesion between the point and tube can be disappointing (Figures 5.18–5.21). Better adhesion can be obtained by using chemically cured composite rather than cyanoacrylate.

## Tube and Hedstroem File Method

This technique described by Suter[17] can be used to remove objects from the root canal. First, space is created around the head of the object that needs to be removed. A tube is then located over it and the two are locked together by gently

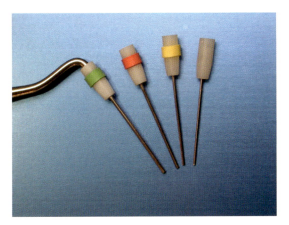

**Figure 5.18**

The Cancellier has a range of different-sized tubes which can be inserted over an object within the root canal. The tubes are held in a handle. This makes their use much easier when operating under a microscope.

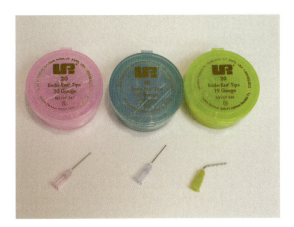

**Figure 5.19**

A cheaper alternative to the Cancellier kit is Endo-Eze tips. These come in different gauges and can be used in a similar manner. The tip of the needle is very malleable and can easily be bent so that the magnified view into the root canal is not obscured.

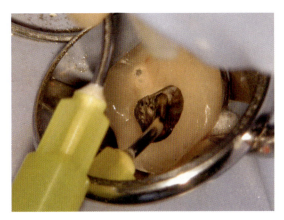

**Figure 5.20**

The Endo-Eze tube is cemented to the fractured instrument using cyanoacrylate glue or chemically cured composite.

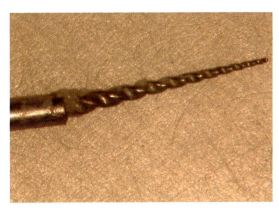

**Figure 5.21**

When the tube and object have bonded together, they can be removed.

screwing a Hedstroem file down the centre of the tube. The technique works well when removing softer materials such as silver points.

*Removing Well-Cemented Silver Points*

Silver points that are well cemented and do not appear to be associated with gross microleakage can be extremely challenging to remove. Any restorative cement material is carefully removed from the pulp chamber using ultrasonics. Retaining the coronal portion of the silver cone will aid removal. An assessment is made under the microscope to find space alongside the cone. A solvent such as Endosolve E or chloroform is used to soften the cement. A small Flexofile (Maillefer, Ballaigues, Switzerland) is then used to try and negotiate a pathway alongside the cone and bypass it. Small amounts of additional solvent may be required. Once a small file (size 10) has been worked alongside the cone, a larger file can be introduced. When a size 15–20 Flexofile is able to pass alongside the silver cone, endosonics can be used to loosen it. Optimistically, the cement will fragment, and by using a gentle filing action the cone will be floated out of the root canal. If the cone appears to be loose but will not lift out of the root canal, then the coronal end

can be grasped with Stieglitz forceps and retrieved. Indirect ultrasonics can be applied to the beaks of the pliers. However, the benefit of this is debatable (Figures 5.22–5.24).

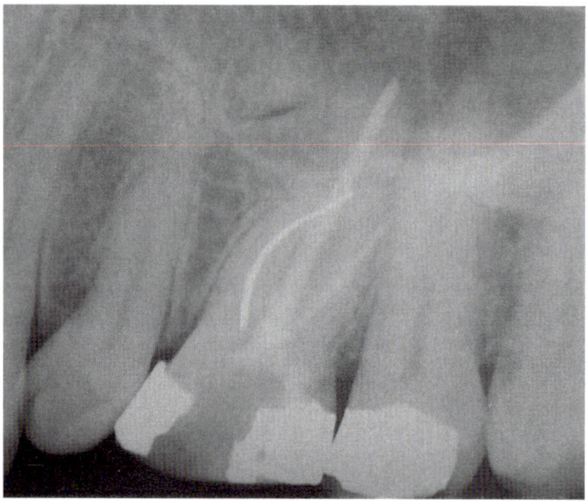

## Sectional Silver Points

When placing a post in the root canal, a sectional silver cone technique was often used. The cone was usually severed 4 or 5 mm from its tip and, after insertion, the apical fragment separated by rotating the coronal portion. In order to remove the apical portion of a sectional silver cone, adequate access and coronal flaring must first be carried out. An

**Figure 5.22**

In this maxillary molar, there was a silver point in the mesial buccal canal. The point had sheared off at orifice level and the root canal was moderately curved. The point was also well cemented. Retrieval in this situation is complex. Space will need to be made alongside the cone so that it can be retrieved. It is useful in the mesiobuccal root of maxillary molars to assess whether there is a second root canal. Sometimes preparing the second mesiobuccal canal will allow the introduction of irrigant to the level of the primary mesiobuccal canal. These canals are often joined by an isthmus. The isthmus will occasionally provide a channel along which small files can be introduced to bypass the cone.

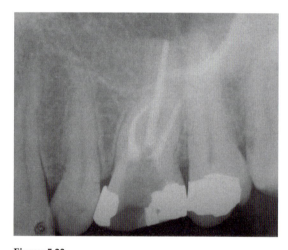

**Figure 5.23**

The cone was retrieved and root canal retreatment carried out in a conventional manner. The root canals were sealed using a vertically compacted gutta percha technique.

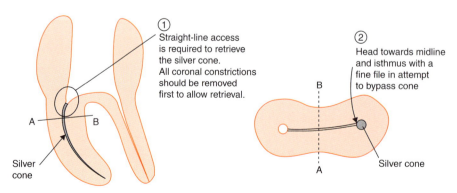

① Straight-line access is required to retrieve the silver cone. All coronal constrictions should be removed first to allow retrieval.

A        B

Silver cone

② Head towards midline and isthmus with a fine file in attempt to bypass cone

B

A        Silver cone

**Figure 5.24**

Removal of silver points.

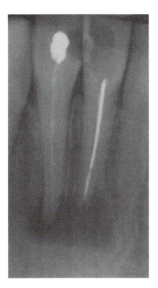

**Figure 5.25**

In this case there is a sectional silver point in the mandibular left central incisor and a single cone gutta percha root filling in the mandibular right central incisor. The teeth are both restorable, have no evidence of periodontal disease and therefore root canal retreatment should have a good prognosis.

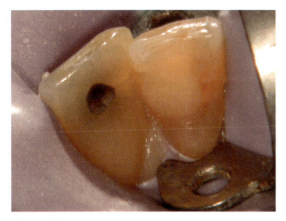

**Figure 5.26**

It can be clearly seen that the access cavities in both mandibular incisors are inadequate and incorrectly positioned. Failing to extend the access in mandibular incisors far enough in the direction of the incisal edge will often lead to inadequate cleaning of the root canal system. It is virtually impossible to engage a lingual canal from this aspect without providing adequate access.

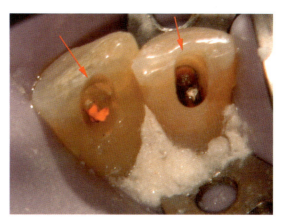

**Figure 5.27**

The access cavities have been modified and now extend from the cingulum to the incisal edge (indicated by red arrows). Good straight-line access to both buccal and lingual canals can now be achieved. The coronal part of the silver point root filling is clearly visible. There is space alongside the cone. The root canal was irrigated with 3% sodium hypochlorite and endosonics inserted alongside the coronal part of the silver point to loosen it.

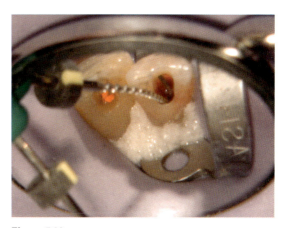

**Figure 5.28**

The silver point was then retrieved by engaging it with a Hedstroem file. When removed, the silver point was retrieved.

estimate of the depth of the piece of silver cone to be removed can be made from a pre-operative paralleling radiograph. The root canal is enlarged to the coronal part of this using conventional nickel–titanium rotary instruments or Gates–Glidden burs. Using an operating microscope, the coronal part of the silver cone can now be visualized. Solvent is

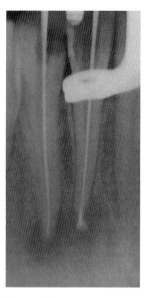

**Figure 5.29**

A diagnostic working length estimation radiograph revealed that the root canals were all patent to the apex. There were only single canals in both mandibular incisors; however, they were biconcave in cross section.

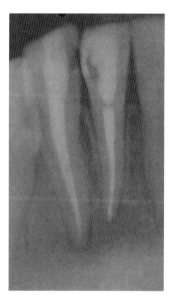

**Figure 5.30**

Following thorough disinfection and the placement of calcium hydroxide as a medicament, the root canals were obturated with a vertically compacted gutta percha technique. The access cavities were sealed with a resin-modified glass ionomer.

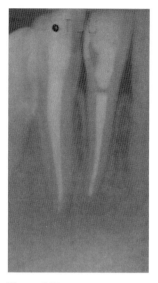

**Figure 5.31**

Six months following obturation, there was good evidence of bony healing. Permanent restorations can now be placed in the access cavities. In this case, a light-cured composite probably offers the simplest solution.

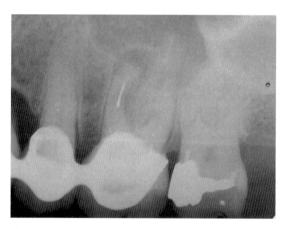

**Figure 5.32**

In the maxillary left first molar, there was an apical silver point in the curved mesiobuccal root. There was a periapical radiolucency associated with this root. The tooth provided a splinted abutment for a long-span anterior bridge. It would not be feasible to section the bridge and carry out root canal retreatment in isolation, as this could jeopardize the survival of the remaining bridge work. In the first instance root canal retreatment should be undertaken to ensure that the root canals are as clean as possible. If it were impossible to retrieve the silver cone, the case would be obturated to the most apical extent. Endodontic surgery would then be considered should symptoms persist or the lesion not heal.

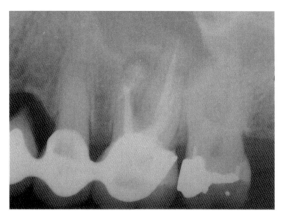

**Figure 5.33**

Due to the angulation and curvature of the mesiobuccal root, a modified access was created and a staging platform created over the coronal aspect of the silver cone. The silver cone was then retrieved using endosonics. Next, the canal was renegotiated, shaped, cleaned and obturated using a vertically compacted gutta technique.

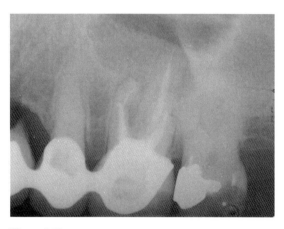

**Figure 5.34**

Six months following root canal retreatment, there was good evidence of bony healing. The tooth was not symptomatic, and therefore the likelihood of surgery being required is extremely slim.

introduced into the canal and a small Flexofile used to try to bypass the fragment. Fortunately, in many teeth the root canal is not circular in cross section but has an oval- or fin- shaped morphology. A good knowledge of dental anatomy will help the operator

ascertain where an attempt at bypassing will be most likely to succeed. Endosonics can also be useful in attempting to create space alongside the silver point. Once space has been created, ultrasonic irrigation with endosonics will generally flush out the small piece of silver point (Figures 5.25–5.34).

## Braiding

Another useful technique for removing small objects from the apical third of the root canals is braiding. Two or more Hedstroem files are inserted alongside the object and then wound together. The intertwined instruments grip the object and, when removed, should retrieve it. This technique can be invaluable for retrieving silver points, fractured instruments, small pieces of gutta percha cone or acrylic points.

## REMOVING SEPARATED INSTRUMENTS

The degree of difficulty when retrieving a separated instrument will depend on the position of the object within the root canal system. Favourable factors for the removal of separated nickel–titanium fragments have been reported to be:

- straight root canals
- anterior teeth
- localization before the curvature in the coronal or mesial third of the root canal
- fragments longer than 5 mm
- hand, as opposed to rotary, instruments.[18,19]

Ideally, any broken instrument that can be visualized with the operating microscope should be removed, and many techniques have been described.[20–24] Fragments that are close to the foramen, protruding beyond it, or hidden from view may require a surgical approach if removal is required. It is important to explain to the patient that a broken instrument itself is not a direct cause of treatment failure. A patient's symptoms or a radiolucency may have persisted because the object has prevented adequate disinfection or elimination of bacteria. Therefore, during retreatment the operator should aim to remove the separated instrument so that the root canal can be thoroughly cleaned and shaped. If this is not possible, then the instrument may be bypassed to allow access to the portion of the root canal that has not been disinfected.

Hedstroem files can be very retentive when broken in root canals, as the blades of the file engage with the dentine of the root canal walls. Spiral fillers can act like a spring and become wedged in the root canal. Pulling a spiral filler in an attempt to retrieve it before adequate loosening can often just result in unwinding of the instrument. Nickel–titanium instruments can become firmly wedged as the instrument attempts to straighten within a curvature in the root canal and this can make retrieval more difficult.

If possible, an assessment of the microbial status of the root canal at the time of the accident is of importance. During treatment of a vital pulp, instrument fracture may be of lesser consequence. There should be little evidence of microbial infection, and therefore the long-term prognosis despite instrument failure should be reasonable. On the other hand, when a tooth has an obvious periapical radiolucency associated with it and the root canal is undoubtedly infected, separation of an instrument early in the preparation sequence may result in the root canal being inadequately cleaned. This is no basis for a predictable outcome. After all, the instrument is not going to provide an effective seal, and the root canal will remain infected.

### Retrieval of Stainless Steel Instruments

If an instrument has fractured coronally and can be bypassed, a small file is first introduced alongside it. Endosonics can then be used to loosen the instrument within the root canal. Alternatively, fine ultrasonic tips such as the CPR 4 and 5 could be used but need a low-power setting to avoid fracture. The aim is to apply ultrasonic energy to the lateral surface of the fractured instrument. If it is applied to the coronal end, this can result in the instrument

embedding itself deeper into the root canal system (Figures 5.35–5.37).

If the instrument has fractured below orifice level, the access and root canal preparation may have to be modified to allow retrieval. Straight-line access is fundamental and allows the creation of an exit pathway for the fractured instrument: in other words, there should be no obstructions to the removal of the instrument.

The access can be modified using a non-end-cutting tungsten carbide bur such as the Endo-Z (Maillefer, Ballaigues, Switzerland) or

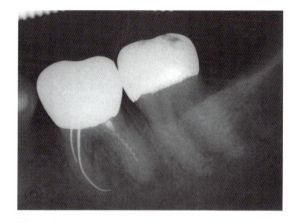

**Figure 5.35**

There was a spiral filler in the distal root of this mandibular molar.

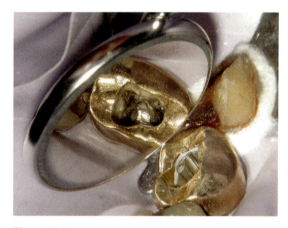

**Figure 5.36**

Access was created using tungsten carbide burs and the spiral filler loosened with an endosonic tip (CPR 5).

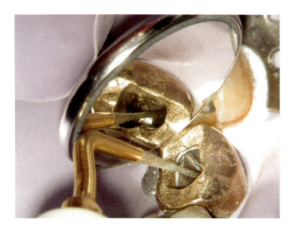

**Figure 5.37**

Ultrasonic vibration loosened the spiral filler sufficiently that it unscrewed itself from the root canal and can be seen on the pulp floor.

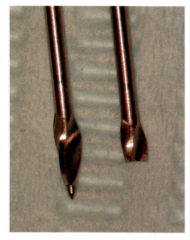

**Figure 5.39**

The non-end-cutting tip of a Gates–Glidden bur can be removed with a long tapered diamond. This creates a very efficient rotary instrument that can be used to create a staging platform over an object that is lodged in the root canal. The modified Gates–Glidden bur must be used with great care and preferably under direct microscopic vision as it is very efficient at cutting.

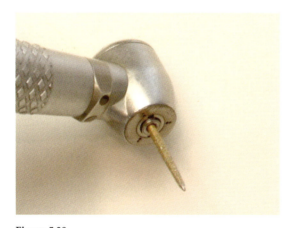

**Figure 5.38**

An LA Axxess bur. This is an excellent instrument for defining the access cavity. The tip is non-end-cutting but pointed and can be inserted into the orifice of the root canal. Applying lateral pressure will refine the lateral borders and create good straight-line access to the root canal system.

an LA Axxess bur (SybronEndo, CA, USA) (Figure 5.38).

The latter is a long-shank diamond bur with a non-cutting but pointed tip. This can be inserted into the orifice of a canal and allows lateral refinement of the access cavity wall. Diamond-coated ultrasonic tips are also useful for refining the access. A Gates–Glidden bur can be modified by removing the safe ended tip (Figure 5.39).

This creates an extremely efficient instrument that will cut a platform over the coronal end of the fractured instrument. Under the operating microscope, space may be visible alongside the instrument into which a small file can be introduced to bypass it. Following this, endosonics are used to try to loosen the fragment and retrieve it. If it does not dislodge, a fine ultrasonic tip can be used to trough around the head of the instrument. Copious irrigation will be required. Packed dentine chips can be removed using a chelating agent such as 17% EDTA (Figures 5.40–5.42).

### The Instrument Removal System

The instrument removal system (IRS) (Dentsply-Maillefer, Ballaigues, Switzerland) is an excellent means of attempting to retrieve the loosened object. This device consists of a hollow tube with a lateral window at the tip.

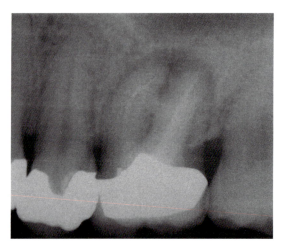

**Figure 5.40**

In this maxillary molar, there was a fractured stainless steel instrument in the mesiobuccal canal. The tooth had periapical radiolucency associated with it and the root canals were undoubtedly infected. The instrument had fractured at the point of curvature of the mesiobuccal canal. Retrieval would be complicated and at best it may only be possible to bypass the instrument, clean the root canal and incorporate it in the root canal filling material. Access was prepared and the root canals flared in the normal manner. The object was retrieved using endosonics. The root canal system could then be cleaned, shaped and disinfected in the normal manner. A second mesiobuccal canal was located and instrumented.

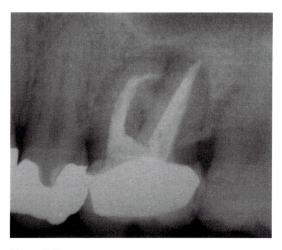

**Figure 5.41**

In this case, a calcium hydroxide/iodoform-based medicament was used to attempt further disinfection of the root canals between visits. A radiograph of the material shows it has been well dispersed in the root canal system.

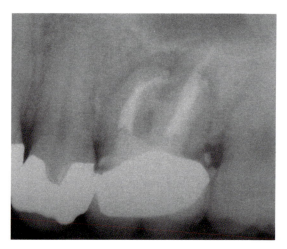

**Figure 5.42**

Following medication for 1 week, the tooth was symptom-free and the buccal sinus tract had healed. The root canals were subsequently obturated with a vertically compacted gutta percha technique and the access sealed with intermediate restorative material (IRM).

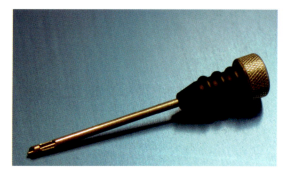

**Figure 5.43**

The instrument removal system (IRS). This consists of a tube with a small window at the tip through which a rod is inserted. The tube is placed over the separated object and, when the rod is inserted and screwed down, it becomes trapped in the window.

A rod is inserted into the tube and the object that is to be removed becomes trapped as the screw is tightened. When engaged, a careful watch-winding action is used to help loosen the instrument and retrieve it from the root canal (Figures 5.43–5.45).[25]

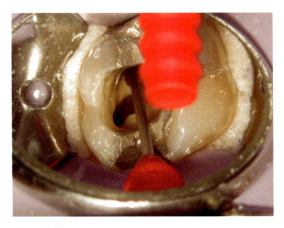

**Figure 5.44**

The instrument removal system (IRS) being used to retrieve a stainless steel instrument from the distobuccal canal of the maxillary molar.

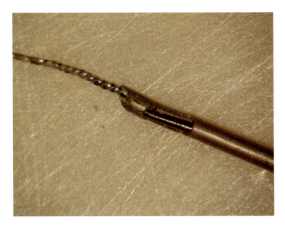

**Figure 5.45**

The fractured instrument has been trapped in the tube. Once engaged, a gentle watch-winding action will often release the object and allow it to be retrieved.

## REMOVAL OF NICKEL–TITANIUM INSTRUMENTS

Nickel–titanium (NiTi) alloys tend to be brittle and removing them with ultrasonics can be frustrating. If the ultrasonic tip touches the head of the fractured file, it will bury itself deeper into the root canal. Excessive use of ultrasonic vibration can result in further fracture of the separated instrument, resulting in an even more difficult retrieval situation.

There are four phases in the retrieval of a fractured nickel–titanium instrument:

- modification of access
- the creation of an adequate exit pathway
- loosening of the instrument
- retrieval.

### Modification of the Access Cavity

A common reason for failure of nickel–titanium rotary instruments is inadequate access preparation. Placement of the access cavity in the incorrect position or making it too small puts unnecessary stress on the instrument as it is rotated in the root canal. The instrument then fails as a result of cyclical fatigue.[26] At the other extreme, too large an access unnecessarily weakens the tooth and may make it more difficult to restore.

When attempting to remove a fractured instrument from a curved canal, any primary curvatures or constrictions need to be removed. This will allow the creation of direct access to the coronal part of the instrument and hence a straight-line exit pathway for retrieval.

### The Exit Pathway

Direct access is created in the root canal coronal to the fractured instrument to allow an unimpeded exit. Modified Gates–Glidden burs are probably the most efficient means of achieving this. This has been described as the creation of a staging platform[27] that allows the use of ultrasonic tips under direct vision with a microscope (Figures 5.46–5.49).

### Loosening

Being careful to avoid intimate contact with the head of the fractured instrument, a fine

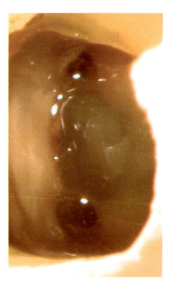

**Figure 5.46**

There was a separated nickel–titanium orifice shaper in the mesiobuccal canal of this mandibular molar. The root canal has been inadequately flared and this is probably why the instrument separated.

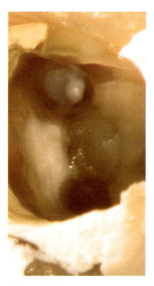

**Figure 5.47**

An exit pathway should be created to the coronal aspect of the fractured object. In this case it was created with Gates–Glidden burs. The canal has deliberately been transported into the bulkiest region of the root canal. A modified Gates–Glidden bur is then used to create a staging platform around the head of the separated instrument.

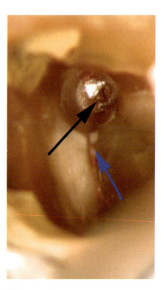

**Figure 5.48**

The staging platform has now been created and there is a small rim of dentine around the fractured instrument. An isthmus can be seen alongside the fractured instrument (indicated by a blue arrow). An initial attempt to bypass the object with small hand files is made where the isthmus runs across the staging platform (indicated by a black arrow). If space can be created, endosonic files or a fine ultrasonic tip can be used to vibrate the object and loosen it. If the object is wedged firmly into the root canal, an ultrasonic tip can be used to trough around the head.

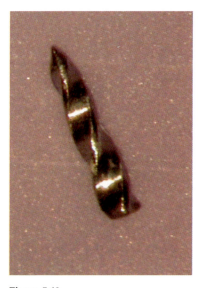

**Figure 5.49**

The instrument tip removed from the previous case.

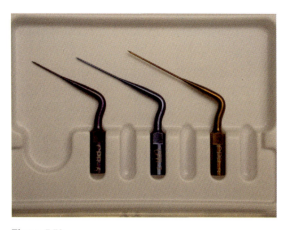

**Figure 5.50**

CPR 6, 7 and 8. These tips are extremely fine and can be used deep into the root canal system with little risk of damage to the root canal. They are a means of applying ultrasonic force to the lateral aspect of an object that may be wedged in the root canal.

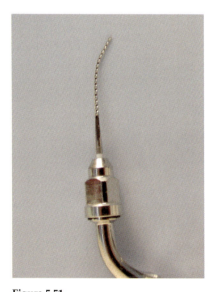

**Figure 5.51**

A modified endosonic tip can be a useful tool for the removal of small objects.

ultrasonic tip such as CPR 6, 7 or 8 can be used to trough around it, creating space (Figure 5.50).

Light pressure can then be applied to the lateral aspect of the fractured instrument with the ultrasonic tip. This will sometimes encourage the rotary file to unscrew. Sometimes space may be limited, and even the finest ultrasonic tip will prove to be too large or obscure the view in the operating microscope. In this situation, an endosonic file can be modified to produce a very fine but relatively robust instrument. The apical 6 mm of an ISO size 15 endosonic file is removed with a pair of scissors, producing an extremely fine micro-instrument that can also be pre-bent to allow better visualization deep in the root canal. It is an efficient tool but should only be used when operating with a microscope (Figure 5.51). Any stainless steel file can be used in this way.

Most nickel–titanium rotary instruments have a cross section consisting of flutes and blades. With direct vision under the operating microscope, the endosonic file, activated at low power, is first placed in the flutes to selectively remove dentine alongside the broken instrument. If this fails to result in any loosening of the fractured instrument, the endosonic file can be used to trough carefully around the head. Following this, lateral placement of the endosonic file against the fractured nickel–titanium instrument is used to help loosen the instrument. Copious irrigation with EDTA is used to clear debris after each short burst of ultrasound. If the instrument cannot be retrieved by ultrasonics alone, a removal system will be required. The IRS is probably one of the most efficient means of retrieving an instrument in this situation. Extractors such as the Masserann or Meitrac are often too cumbersome for use in intricate root canals. Often, the separated instrument cannot easily be retrieved because it is flexing within the curved root canal and pressing against the outer wall. The tube of an IRS extractor has a bevelled tip and this can be very helpful to scoop the flexed nickel–titanium fragment into it. Engaging the rod and screwing both halves together will grip the instrument. Careful watch-winding and anti-clockwise rotation should then result in retrieval (Figures 5.52–5.68).

## Bypassing

If it is not possible to retrieve an instrument or the operator feels that the risk of perforation

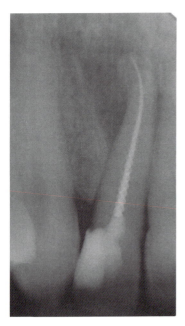

**Figure 5.52**

In this maxillary lateral incisor, a nickel–titanium Profile instrument has separated. The entire working length is present in the root canal system. Retrieval of an instrument fragment such as this should be relatively simple, as it is most likely to be binding coronally.

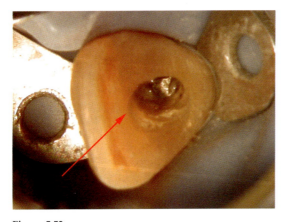

**Figure 5.53**

The access cavity is first modified so that straight-line access to the head of the instrument can be achieved and the instrument has a clear exit pathway for retrieval. A red arrow indicates extension of the access cavity onto the incisal edge. A fine ultrasonic tip, such as the CPR 2, 3 or CT4, is used to apply ultrasonic force to the lateral aspect of the Profile.

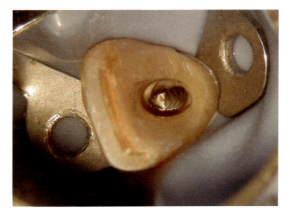

**Figure 5.54**

Following irrigation and ultrasonic vibration, the Profile is unscrewed from the root canal. It is now situated in the access cavity and can be easily retrieved with a pair of Stieglitz forceps.

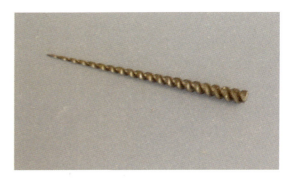

**Figure 5.55**

The Profile instrument removed intact.

or irreversible damage is too great, then bypassing should be attempted. In this way, the root canal beyond the fractured instrument can be cleaned in the normal manner and the fractured instrument is incorporated in the root canal filling. The technique for bypassing an instrument is similar to that for retrieving silver cones or fractured instruments. A good knowledge of anatomy is useful. For example, in the mesial canals of mandibular molars there is often an isthmus in the apical third.[28] Directing a fine file towards the centre line of the tooth may

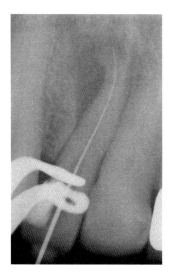

**Figure 5.56**

A diagnostic working length radiograph showed that the root canal was patent to the apex. The apical region had been over-prepared and possibly resorbed as a result of chronic inflammation. The canal was tapered using nickel–titanium rotary instruments keeping 0.5 mm short of the full working length to avoid further damage to the apical terminus.

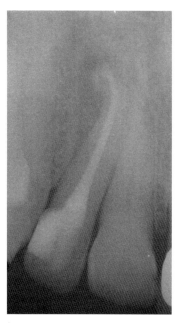

**Figure 5.58**

The case 6 months following obturation shows some evidence of bony healing and absorption of the extruded material.

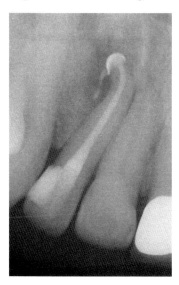

**Figure 5.57**

Following medication with an iodoform-based material the root canal system was obturated with a vertically compacted gutta percha technique because the apical constriction had been over-prepared, zipped and transported. A small amount of medicament and sealer was extruded during the obturation sequence. This should be absorbed over a few months.

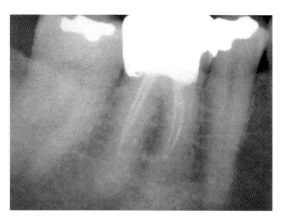

**Figure 5.59**

In this mandibular molar, the root canal system had been poorly root filled. The tooth was symptomatic. There were single cone root fillings in the mesial and distal root canals. None of the canals had been prepared adequately. There was a separated nickel–titanium instrument in the mesiobuccal canal. This was situated in the mid-third around a curvature. Retrieval would be complicated and bypassing it would offer the next best alternative.

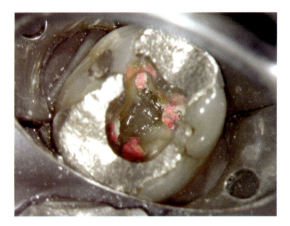

**Figure 5.60**

An access cavity was made that provided good straight-line access to all the root canals. The gutta percha and sealer can be seen in the coronal orifices of the four root canals. The pulp floor is much darker than the walls of the access and the pulp floor map clearly shows the four root canals. Gutta percha was removed with Gates–Glidden burs and Hedstroem files. Coronal flaring was then carried out with nickel–titanium rotary instruments. In the mesiobuccal canal, a staging platform was created using a modified Gates–Glidden bur.

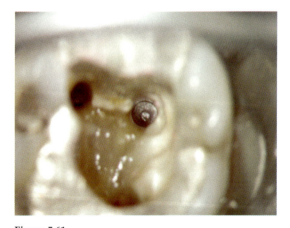

**Figure 5.61**

The head of the instrument can be visualized midway down the root canal surrounded by a rim of dentine.

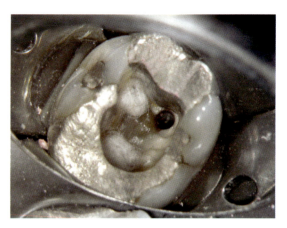

**Figure 5.62**

Before attempting retrieval, cotton wool pellets were placed in the orifices of the other canals to prevent the object being dislodged into them. Ultrasonic energy from a modified endosonic file was then used to loosen the fragment and retrieve it from the root canal.

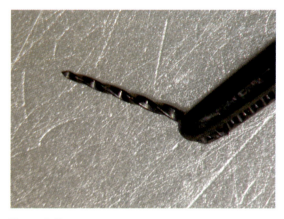

**Figure 5.63**

The instrument as retrieved from the root canal.

enable the isthmus to be engaged and the fractured instrument to be bypassed. In maxillary first molars, there is often a second mesiobuccal canal, which can sometimes be used as a means of bypassing an instrument that has been fractured in the primary mesiobuccal canal. This is especially true if the two canals converge and exit via one orifice. Good radiographic technique, knowledge of root canal anatomy and sensitive tactile feedback will all aid the operator in ascertaining whether this is likely to be achieved.

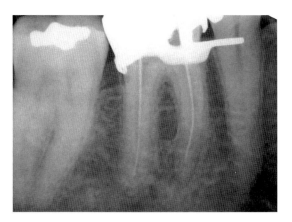

**Figure 5.64**

A diagnostic working length estimation radiograph revealed that all the root canals were patent and could be instrumented to their full extent. Fortunately, the mesial canals had not been ledged and could therefore be renegotiated relatively easily.

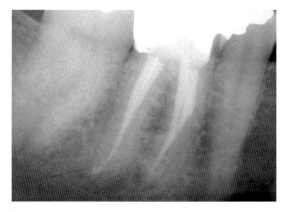

**Figure 5.65**

The case was obturated using a vertically compacted gutta percha technique and the access cavity sealed with a resin-modified glass ionomer. There is a small ledge on the mesiobuccal canal where the staging platform was created. However, retrieval of the fractured instrument has been carried out conservatively and without damaging or perforating the root of the tooth.

## Retaining the Fractured Instrument

If it proves impossible to retrieve or bypass the instrument, there is no alternative but to leave it within the root canal system. The root filling is completed to the most coronal part of

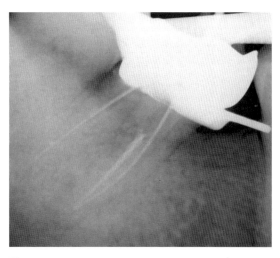

**Figure 5.66**

In this mandibular molar, a greater taper instrument has separated in one of the mesial canals. Retrieval will be complicated due to the angulation of the tooth. Hand files have been inserted in the other canals and show that they are patent. In the mesial root the two canals join at the apex. Straight-line access was created to the level of the fractured instrument and ultrasonic force applied using a modified endosonic tip.

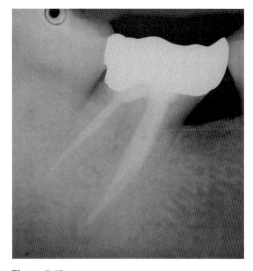

**Figure 5.67**

In this case, a greater amount of dentine had to be removed in order to achieve the objective. There was no risk of perforation. However, treatment was considerably more complicated than in the previous case.

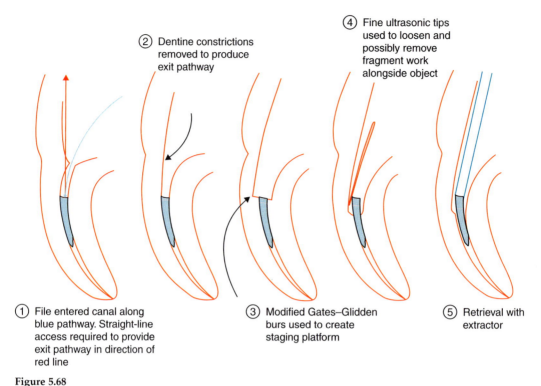

② Dentine constrictions
removed to produce
exit pathway

④ Fine ultrasonic tips
used to loosen and
possibly remove
fragment work
alongside object

① File entered canal along
blue pathway. Straight-line
access required to provide
exit pathway in direction of
red line

③ Modified Gates–Glidden
burs used to create
staging platform

⑤ Retrieval with
extractor

**Figure 5.68**

Removal of nickel–titanium instrument.

the fractured object and the canal obturated. A review is carried out in the normal manner and, if symptoms fail to resolve, then an alternative treatment approach may be required. In teeth without periapical radiolucency, this should not appear to affect the prognosis.[29,30]

## REFERENCES

1. Carr GB. Microscopes in endodontics. *Journal of the Californian Dental Association* 1992; **20:** 55–61.
2. Hülsmann M, Schinkel I. Influence of several factors on the success or failure of removal of fractured instruments from the root canal. *Endodontics and Dental Traumatology* 1999; **15:** 252–258.
3. Ward JR, Parashos P, Messer HH. Evaluation of an ultrasonic technique to remove fractured rotary nickel-titanium instruments from root canals: an experimental study. *Journal of Endodontics* 2003; **29:** 756–763.
4. Suter B, Lussi A, Sequiera P. Probability of removing fractured instruments from root canals. *International Endodontic Journal* 2005; **38:** 112–123.
5. Ritchie GM, Weine FS, Smulson MH. Modifications for successful use of silver points in endodontics. *Journal of the Academy of General Dentistry* 1972; **20:** 35–39.
6. Weine FS, Healey HJ, Lippert JL. Use of silver points with improved digital control. *Journal American Dental Association* 1971; **83:** 125–128.
7. Chana H, Briggs P, Moss R. Degradation of a silver point in association with endodontic infection. *International Endodontic Journal* 1998; **31:** 141–146.
8. Goon WW, Lugassy AA. Periapical electrolytic corrosion in the failure of silver

point endodontic restorations: report of two cases. *Quintessence International* 1995; **26:** 629–633.

9. Brady JM, del Rio CE. Corrosion of endodontic silver cones in humans: a scanning electron microscope and X-ray microprobe study. *Journal of Endodontics* 1975; **1:** 205–210.

10. Goldberg F. Relation between corroded silver points and endodontic failures. *Journal of Endodontics* 1981; **7:** 224–227.

11. Plack WF, Vire DE. Retrieval of endodontic silver points. *General Dentistry* 1984; **32:** 124–127.

12. Crane DL. Posts, points, and instruments: how to retrieve them, Part 1. *Compendium* 1990; **11:** 563–565.

13. Hülsmann M. The retrieval of silver cones using different techniques. *International Endodontic Journal* 1990; **23:** 130–134.

14. Coutinho Filho T, Krebs RL, Berlinck TC, Galindo RG. Retrieval of a broken endodontic instrument using cyanoacrylate adhesive. Case report. *Brazilian Dental Journal* 1998; **9:** 57–60.

15. Spriggs K, Gettleman B, Messer HH. Evaluation of a new method for silver point removal. *Journal of Endodontics* 1990; **16:** 335–338.

16. Elazer PD, O'Connor RP. Innovative uses of hypodermic needles in endodontics. *Journal of Endodontics* 1999; **25:** 190–191.

17. Suter B. A new method for retrieving silver points and separated instruments from root canals. *Journal of Endodontics* 1998; **24:** 446–448.

18. Shen Y, Peng B, Cheung GS. Factors associated with the removal of fractured NiTi instruments from root canals. *Oral Surgery, Oral Medicine, Oral Pathology, Oral Radiology, Endodontics* 2004; **98:** 605–610.

19. Hülsmann M, Schinkel I. Influence of several factors on the success or failure of removal of fractured instruments from the root canal. *Endodontics and Dental Traumatology* 1999; **15:** 252–258.

20. Souyave LC, Inglis AT, Alcalay M. Removal of fractured endodontic instruments using ultrasonics. *British Dental Journal* 1985; **159:** 251–253.

21. Hülsmann M. Removal of fractured instruments using a combined automated/ ultrasonic technique. *Journal of Endodontics* 1994; **20:** 144–147.

22. McCullock AJ. The removal of restorations and foreign objects from root canals. *Quintessence International* 1993; **24:** 245–249.

23. Hülsmann M. Methods for removing metal obstructions from the root canal. *Endodontics and Dental Traumatolology* 1993; **9:** 223–237.

24. Nagai O, Tagi N, Kayaba Y, Kodama S, Osada T. Ultrasonic removal of broken instruments in root canals. *International Endodontic Journal* 1986; **19:** 298–304.

25. Ruddle CJ. Removal of broken instruments. *Endodontic Practice* 2003; **6:** 13–19.

26. Haikel Y, Serfaty R, Bateman G, Senger B, Alleman C. Dynamic and cyclic fatigue of engine-driven rotary nickel-titanium instruments. *Journal of Endodontics* 1999; **25:** 434–440.

27. Ward JR, Parashos P, Messer HH. Evaluation of an ultrasonic technique to remove fractured rotary nickel-titanium endodontic instruments from root canals: clinical cases. *Journal of Endodontics* 2003; **29:** 764–767.

28. von Arx T. Frequency and type of canal isthmuses in first molars detected by endoscopic inspection during periradicular surgery. *International Endodontic Journal* 2005; **38:** 160–168.

29. Grossman LI. Fate of endodontically treated teeth with fractured instruments. *Journal of the British Endodontic Society* 1968; **2:** 35–37.

30. Crump MC, Natkin E. Relationship of broken root canal instruments to endodontic case prognosis: a clinical investigation. *Journal of the American Dental Association* 1970; **80:** 1341–1347.

# 6 PERFORATION REPAIR AND RENEGOTIATING THE ROOT CANAL SYSTEM FOLLOWING DISMANTLING

**CONTENTS • Introduction • Preventing Perforation • Important Factors in Dealing with Perforations • Furcation Perforation • Materials • Perforation Repair Technique • Strip Perforation Repair • Post Space Perforation Repair • Perforation Repair in the Apical Region • Renegotiating the Root Canal Following Dismantling • References**

## INTRODUCTION

Perforation can occur during the preparation of an access cavity, the root canals, post space preparation or rarely as the result of expansion of an inflammatory resorption defect. Using an operating microscope and modern endodontic techniques, many cases that would have previously required a surgical approach or extraction can be treated non-surgically.

## PREVENTING PERFORATION

Perforation of the furcation can be prevented by careful planning and treatment. A paralleling radiograph gives a good indication of the depth of the pulp floor and can be used to estimate the depth at which burs will penetrate the pulp chamber. The pulp floor map is used to locate root canal orifices (Figure 6.1).

If the canals are sclerosed or hidden, small increments of dentine are removed under microscopic illumination and a confirmatory radiograph taken to confirm orientation if there is any doubt. An apex locator and radiograph are used to estimate root canal length. This is confirmed with a paralleling radiograph and should match the operator's expected length from knowledge of root canal anatomy. During preparation, Gates–Glidden burs should be used conservatively. They should not penetrate too deeply and smaller sizes are recommended

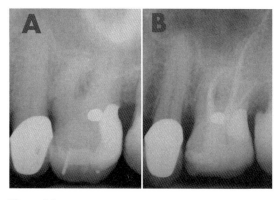

**Figure 6.1**

(A) A maxillary molar that requires root canal treatment. There has been significant irritation dentine formed in response to bacterial leakage around extensive restorations. The pulp chamber roof and floor are in very close proximity. It would be easy to accidentally perforate the furcation during access cavity preparation. Careful measurement from the preoperative radiograph, magnification and illumination all allow the operator to prepare an access confidently without risk. (B) The completed case.

in curved canals where a strip perforation may occur. The operator should try to direct the cutting action into the bulkiest wall of dentine, which also helps straighten the first curvature of the root canal and improves straight-line access. Non-landed rotary instruments should not be overused. They will cut laterally and can subsequently perforate. Likewise, large rotary instruments used for coronal flaring can strip perforate if used too deeply. Irrigating solutions keep the dentine chips that are created during preparation in suspension and prevent blocking. If dentine chips are packed into the apical region of the root canal, the preparation can become transported internally, which could lead to apical perforation. When preparing a post hole, a Gates–Glidden bur should be used to prepare a pilot hole before using post drills. The post drills should be used with coolant and the diameter gradually increased. Preparation of post holes under direct vision with a microscope can prevent transportation and perforation.

## IMPORTANT FACTORS IN DEALING WITH PERFORATIONS

Four factors are considered when dealing with perforations.[1]

### Level

A perforation above the alveolar bone level can usually be treated as a restorative problem using conventional filling techniques. Defects that are below the crestal bone level can often be treated non-surgically using the techniques described in this chapter. Perforations that have occurred at the level of the crestal bone and have direct communication via the periodontal ligament or a periodontal pocket to the oral cavity can be complex to treat. There is a high risk of microleakage in this situation and the repair may result in a persistent periodontal pocket following treatment due to the development of subgingival plaque being promoted by the rough surface of the repair material.[2]

### Location

Perforations that have damaged the root canal orifice and pulp floor can be more difficult to seal. Access to the lingual surface of the root may not be feasible if a surgical approach for repair is proposed.

### Size

The larger the perforation, the greater the surface area that will need to be sealed.

### Time

It is always preferable to seal a perforation as soon as possible, since there is less likelihood of microleakage, infection or major bone resorption having occurred.

## FURCATION PERFORATION

### Micro-Perforation (< 0.5 mm)

Small perforations of the pulp floor can be conveniently sealed using light-cured composites or resin-modified glass ionomer.

The pulp floor is disinfected using sodium hypochlorite and EDTA. The area over the perforation is either acid-etched with phosphoric acid and then restored with conventional flowable composite or conditioned and restored with a resin-modified glass ionomer (Figures 6.2, 6.3).

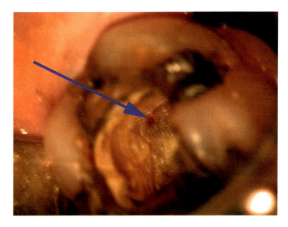

**Figure 6.2**

In this mandibular molar, a micro-perforation has been made in the wall of the access cavity indicated by a blue arrow. In this situation, the perforation can be cleaned with sodium hypochlorite and sealed very effectively with a glass ionomer or light-cured composite.

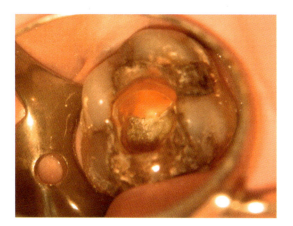

**Figure 6.3**

The micro-perforation was simply sealed with a glass ionomer.

## Larger Perforations (> 0.5 mm)

If there is little evidence of infection, granulation tissue or osseous resorption, the repair material can be packed directly into the perforation site following disinfection. If there has been bony resorption and a significant osseous defect is present, a matrix may be required before placement of the repair material.

## MATERIALS

There are many materials that have been suggested for use in repairing perforations. Some are also utilized as root-end filling material in surgical endodontics. It would seem sensible to use a material for perforation repair that has been shown to be biocompatible and that works well in the surgical environment, especially when the material will be in close proximity to the alveolar bone.

There are three materials that are in common use:

- mineral trioxide aggregate (ProRoot MTA, Dentsply-Maillefer, Ballaigues, Switzerland)
- ethoxybenzoic acid (Super EBA, Staident International, Staines, UK)
- intermediate restorative material (IRM, Dentsply DeTrey, Konstanz, Germany).

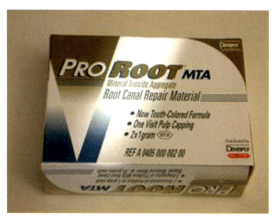

**Figure 6.4**

Mineral trioxide aggregate (MTA) has been shown to be highly biocompatible and an excellent material for the repair of some perforations. It tends to be best suited to the repair of defects which are lined by an osseous crypt and where sufficient bulk of material can be placed. MTA is not ideally suited for the repair of very small perforations.

## Mineral Trioxide Aggregate

MTA has been recommended as a root-end filling material[3] and for the repair of perforations.[4–6] It has excellent biocompatibility[7] when compared with other root-end filling materials. Formation of a new cementum layer has been shown when MTA has been used to repair perforations.[6] The material is able to set and form a seal even in the presence of water or blood.[4,8] MTA comes as a powder and is mixed with sterile water to a slurry consistency. It can be a difficult material to handle, has a long setting time (2 hours 45 minutes) and normally requires a two-visit approach for perforation repair. Radiographically, the material appears slightly more opaque than gutta percha (Figure 6.4).

## Super Ethoxybenzoic Acid

Super EBA is a modified form of zinc oxide–eugenol cement. Orthobenzoic acid forms part of the liquid component and aluminium

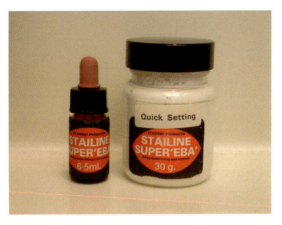

**Figure 6.5**

Super EBA (ethoxybenzoic acid) has been used for root-end surgery for many years and can be used to repair perforations. It will work well in smaller cavities.

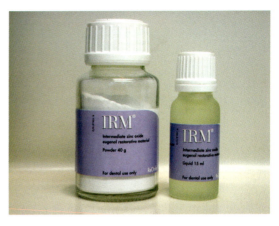

**Figure 6.6**

Intermediate restorative material (IRM) is a reinforced zinc oxide–eugenol material that can be used for perforation repair.

oxide is added to the powder. The material has a neutral pH and low solubility. It will adhere to dentine in the presence of moisture or blood contamination[8] and periapical tissue repair has been demonstrated when it has been used as a root-end filling.[9] EBA cement has a relatively short working time and tends to adhere well to most surfaces. It can therefore be difficult to handle. The material has similar radio-opacity to gutta percha (Figure 6.5).

### Intermediate Restorative Material

IRM is a reinforced zinc oxide–eugenol cement. It has been used as a root-end filling material with good results.[10] Indeed, in a recent prospective study comparing MTA and IRM as root-end filling materials, there was no significant difference in success rates at 2 years.[11] When used in root-end surgery the material is mixed with a high powder/liquid ratio to reduce the irritant effects of the eugenol, increase setting time, enhance placement and reduce dissolution in tissue fluid.[12] It has a good working time and is radio-opaque (Figure 6.6).

## PERFORATION REPAIR TECHNIQUE

### Single Stage

The perforation site is cleaned and disinfected using sodium hypochlorite. The solution is not injected through the perforation but allowed to bathe the area and pulp chamber. Ultrasonics can be used to debride the edges of the perforation site if required. The perforation is finally rinsed with a 0.2% solution of chlorhexidine gluconate before being dried with large paper points or a Stropko irrigator tip. Materials such as IRM or Super EBA are mixed and packed directly into the defect.

If there has been significant bony resorption, a matrix may be required to fill the defect before packing the perforation repair material. Absorbable bovine collagen (CollaCote, Calcitek, USA) can be cut into small pieces and packed into the bony lesion until a solid barrier is established at the external root canal wall. The perforation repair material can be packed directly onto the matrix (Figures 6.7–6.14).

### Two Stages

As MTA has a long setting time, a two-stage procedure will be required. The perforation

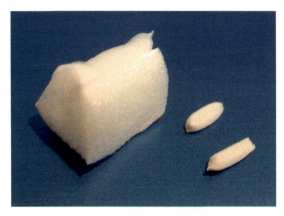

**Figure 6.7**

A haemostat material can be used to create a matrix onto which repair material is packed.

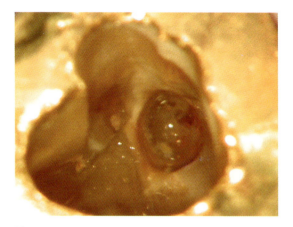

**Figure 6.9**

The root canal orifice has been identified and the access cavity modified so that it can be repaired. The defect has been cleaned with 4% sodium hypochlorite and EDTA.

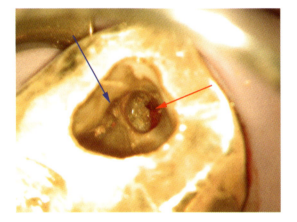

**Figure 6.8**

In this mandibular molar, a large perforation has been created in the wall of the access chamber. This is supracrestal but at the level of the gingival tissues. (The red arrow indicates perforation, the blue arrow the position of the canal orifice.)

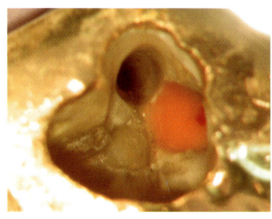

**Figure 6.10**

The defect has been filled with a resin-modified glass ionomer.

site is cleaned in the same manner as described previously. The root canals can either be permanently obturated or filled with calcium hydroxide. Once the site has been cleaned, an assessment is made to ascertain whether a matrix is required. MTA has excellent biocompatibility and can be packed directly into a bony defect. This may not look as tidy on a radiograph, but biologically should not affect healing and will provide a good seal. If a matrix is required, then Collecote can be used. MTA is packed into the defect and sealed into the access chamber using a damp pellet and IRM. If the canals have been obturated, then MTA can also be packed across the pulp floor in some instances.

At a second visit 48 hours later, the access is reopened and the MTA probed to check that it has hardened. The access cavity can be permanently sealed (Figures 6.15–6.19).

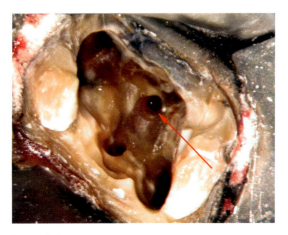

**Figure 6.11**

In this maxillary molar, there is a perforation adjacent to the distobuccal canal (red arrow). The root canals have been cleaned, shaped and medicament placed for 1 week. Following further irrigation, the perforation can be repaired.

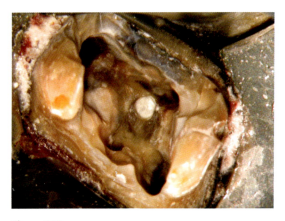

**Figure 6.12**

The defect in this case was repaired with IRM. Material has been plugged into the perforation site and burnished.

## STRIP PERFORATION REPAIR

A strip perforation can be caused by over-use of Gates–Glidden burs or rotary coronal flaring instruments. The resultant defect is a narrow slit-like perforation on the internal curvature of the root canal. A strip perforation can be detected using an apex locator but will be easier to repair if it is visible under the operating microscope.

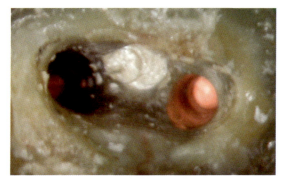

**Figure 6.13**

In this maxillary premolar, a furcal perforation has been created during post preparation. This has subsequently been sealed with Super EBA.

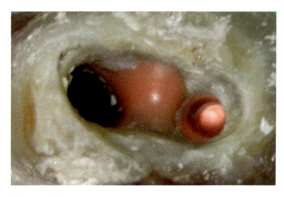

**Figure 6.14**

The Super EBA material has been covered with a coating of resin-modified glass ionomer.

Preparation and cleaning are completed in the usual manner using irrigants such as sodium hypochlorite and EDTA. Endosonics can also be useful for delivering irrigant. The solutions should percolate into the strip perforation and bathe the defect. It is very important that irrigant is delivered passively and that the solutions are not injected through the perforation and into the bony crypt. Following cleaning, the canal is dried, and in most instances a medicament such as calcium hydroxide is packed into it. At a second appointment, the medicament is washed out of the root canal system using sodium hypochlorite and EDTA. The canal is dried

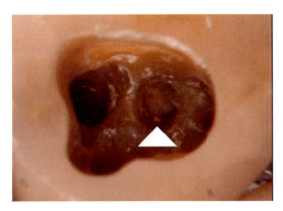

**Figure 6.15**

A large perforation has been made through the furcation of this mandibular molar. The bony crypt can be seen through the perforation site. The root canals have all been instrumented and thoroughly irrigated with sodium hypochlorite.

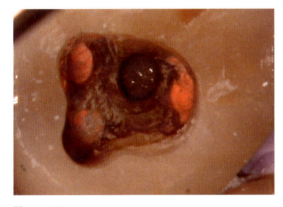

**Figure 6.16**

This large defect is ideally suited to repair with MTA. The material is mixed and then placed into the area. Because MTA is highly biocompatible, it can be placed directly onto the bony surface. However, if there is a large void under the furcation, a reasorbable matrix would normally be packed into it, onto which the MTA material can be placed.

with paper points. If a small plugger can be inserted to within 3 mm of the working length, MTA can be used to obturate the entire canal and, in doing so, the defect will be sealed. If the apical region is too small or inaccessible due to excessive curvature, it is obturated with gutta percha and sealer and then finished just apical to the strip perforation. The remainder of the canal is then packed

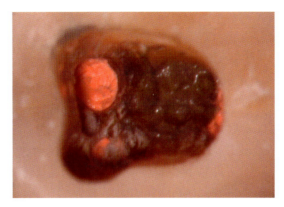

**Figure 6.17**

MTA was then placed across the entire pulp floor to achieve a good seal.

with MTA. A damp pellet or sponge is sealed into the access with IRM. At a further visit it is confirmed that the MTA has set (Figure 6.20).

When obturating a root canal with MTA, it is worthwhile taking a radiograph before sealing the access cavity to check that the material has been positioned correctly. If it is short or there are voids present, the material can easily be removed by irrigating with sterile saline or local anaesthetic and the canal repacked. Another technique for obturating the entire canal involves mixing the MTA slightly wetter than usual and placing it into the root canal. A short burst of ultrasound transmitted through it with an endosonic file causes the MTA to slump into the root canal.

## POST SPACE PERFORATION REPAIR

It is preferable that the perforation site is visible with the operating microscope and accessible to instrumentation. The previous restoration is dismantled and the root canal cleaned with irrigants. The perforation should be cleaned passively with irrigant solutions. There is often granulation tissue present in the defect, and this has to be displaced to allow the placement of perforation repair material.

Lemon[13] introduced the 'internal matrix concept' for the treatment of such root perforations. In this technique hydroxyapatite used as the external matrix and the defect was filled

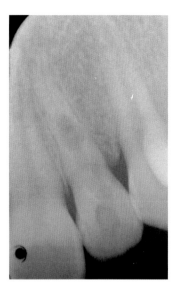

**Figure 6.18**

In this maxillary lateral incisor, there is a perforation below crestal bone level. The tooth has also suffered from internal resorption.

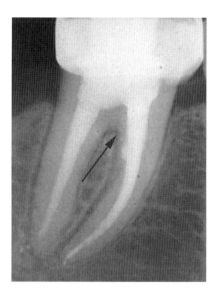

**Figure 6.20**

In this case, a strip perforation had been created in the mesial canals during over-use of nickel–titanium rotary instruments (arrow). The apical portion of the root canal was obturated with gutta percha and the coronal part sealed with MTA. This will also seal the strip perforation defect.

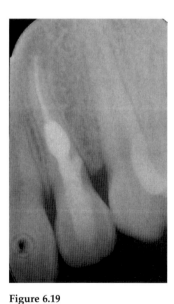

**Figure 6.19**

The root canal has been obturated using the vertically compacted gutta percha technique and thermoplasticized Obtura gutta percha. The perforation has been repaired with MTA. (Radiograph courtesy of James Aquilina.)

with amalgam. The technique has been modified for use with MTA. Because MTA does not require a firm barrier like amalgam to pack against, a resorbable collagen matrix can be used.

Collecote is packed through the defect and used to push any granulation tissue extraradicularly. MTA can then be placed into the defect with an MTA gun (Dentsply-Maillefer, Ballaigues, Switzerland) or picked up on a plugger tip and packed into place. Direct visualization is important to prevent material occluding the root canal space. This technique has been shown to be effective in clinical use.[14] If the defect cannot be visualized, a surgical approach may be more effective (Figures 6.21–6.24).

## PERFORATION REPAIR IN THE APICAL REGION

A micro-perforation, perhaps caused by an instrumentation error, can usually be sealed using conventional obturation techniques. The

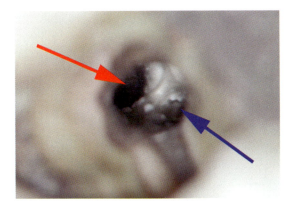

**Figure 6.21**

The root canal of this tooth has been perforated. (Red arrow indicates the position of the perforation, the blue arrow shows the root canal.)

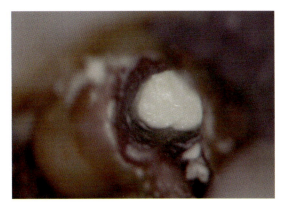

**Figure 6.23**

MTA has been used to seal the perforation site and the coronal aspect of the root canal.

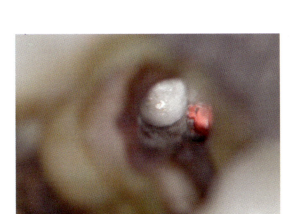

**Figure 6.22**

Matrix material has been plugged through the perforation into the bony defect. The root canal has been sealed with gutta percha.

root canal system is cleaned in the usual manner, dried and obturated with gutta percha and sealer.

If the root canal is relatively straight and the perforation site can be located, obturating the canal with MTA may be feasible. This can be a useful technique for teeth that are to be restored with a post crown, as it can sometimes be difficult to place sufficient gutta percha and sealer to provide an adequate seal. Sometimes, a surgical approach may be required (Figure 6.25).

## RENEGOTIATING THE ROOT CANAL FOLLOWING DISMANTLING

Irritation dentine, pulp stones and other calcifications may make the location of root canal orifices or negotiation of a root canal difficult.

### Exposing the Canal Orifices

Microscopic magnification and illumination combined with ultrasonic tips are invaluable in this situation and provide the most predictable means of locating canal orifices.[15] Ultrasonics allow the precise removal of dentine from the pulp floor with minimal risk of perforation. Ultrasonic diamond-coated tips can be used dry in intermittent bursts to remove dentine. The assistant uses a Stropko irrigator to puff away dentine chips. A solution of 17% EDTA is excellent for clearing the area under exploration. The pulp chamber should be flooded with EDTA solution for 2 minutes. Dentine chips and other debris can then be washed away with sodium hypochlorite. The pulp floor is explored with a DG16 probe or micro-debrider to locate the canal orifices. If the canal is very fine, highly curved or sclerosed, then a fine hand instrument such as a C+ file (Dentsply-Maillefer, Ballaigues, Switzerland) can be used to gauge a pathway.

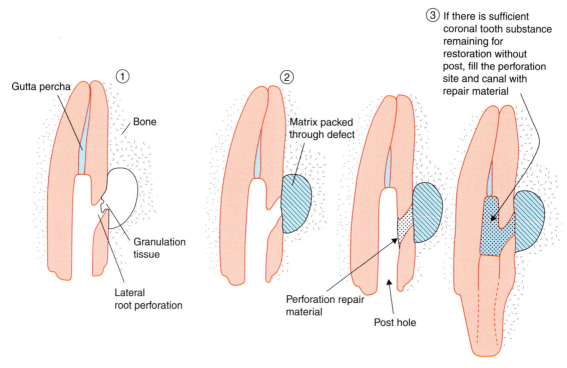

**Figure 6.24**

Internal matrix perforation repair.

A thorough knowledge of the anatomy of the pulp floor and the likely location of the canal orifices is essential. The pulp floor map and the relationship of the floor to surrounding tooth structure should give some idea of the location of root canals (Figures 6.26, 6.27).

The pulp floor tends to be darker than the walls. Dyes, such as iodine in potassium iodide or methylene blue, have been used to demonstrate the location of canal orifices (Figure 6.28).

The orifices tend to be located at an imaginary point directly apical to the original location of the cusp tip. Dentine needs to be removed very carefully when attempting to locate sclerosed canals. Ultrasonic tips such as the CPR 2 and 3 allow precise removal of dentine from the floor of the pulp chamber. Swan-necked LN burs can also be very useful.

If the canal is completely sclerosed for several millimetres apical to the pulp floor,

instruments should be advanced gradually and a confirmatory radiograph exposed to ascertain orientation of the instrument within the canal. Under the microscope, it is often possible to distinguish between irritation dentine occluding the original canal and that of the root wall. The area that needs to be removed tends to be darker (Figure 6.29).

## The Location of Canals in Specific Situations

### The Second Mesiobuccal Canal of Maxillary Molars

Approximately 60% of maxillary molars have two mesiobuccal canals. The orifice of the second mesiobuccal canal (MBII) often lies under a lip of dentine on the mesial wall (Figure 6.30).

There may be two separate orifices but occasionally the MBII branches off the primary

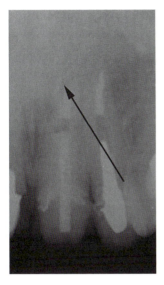

**Figure 6.25**

In this maxillary central incisor, there was a possibility that the root canal had been perforated by previous post space preparation. Because the root canal was very large, it was decided to obturate the apical region with MTA, which will seal any potential perforation (arrow).

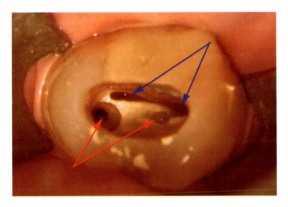

**Figure 6.26**

The pulp floor map has not been used in a previous attempt to find the root canals (blue arrows indicate canal orifices). The bur holes made in attempt to locate the orifices are off-centre (red arrows). Direct vision with the operating microscope makes the mistake look obvious and reinforces the benefit of magnification and illumination for better visualization.

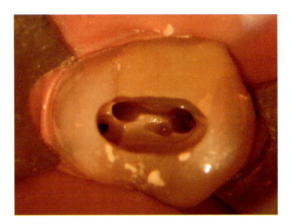

**Figure 6.27**

The correct orifices have now been accessed and flared.

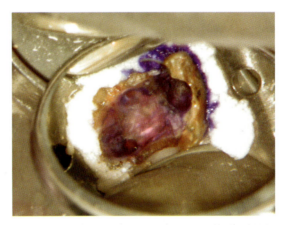

**Figure 6.28**

An indicator dye such as Canal Blue (Dentsply, Weybridge, Surrey, UK) has been used to identify orifices of any remaining root canals in this maxillary molar.

canal just below the pulp floor. When two canals are present, an isthmus will often communicate between them.[16] This can be traced from the primary mesiobuccal canal until the second orifice is located. An estimation for the location of the MBII orifice can be made by visualizing a point at the intersection between a line running from the mesiobuccal to palatal canal and a perpendicular from the distobuccal canal. Dentine is removed in this area using an ultrasonic tip, CPR 2 or 3, or LN bur. When using a microscope under high power, it is useful to scan the entire pulp floor occasionally at a lower magnification to ensure relative positioning and prevent perforation.

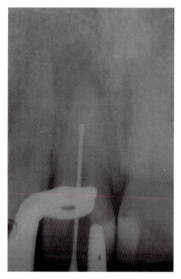

**Figure 6.29**

When attempting to locate a sclerosed root canal using a rotary instrument, a check radiograph is taken to ensure that the instrument is heading in the correct direction.

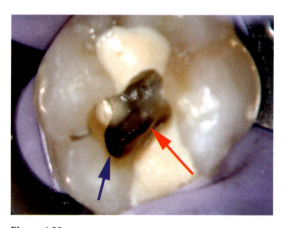

**Figure 6.30**

Troughing between the primary mesiobuccal canal and palatal canal and removing the lip of dentine in this area will often indicate the presence of a second mesiobuccal canal. There is commonly an isthmus between the two, which can be traced.

## Four Canals in Mandibular Molars

Four canals are found in approximately 38% of mandibular molars. If the distal canal does not lie in the midline of the tooth, a second distal canal should be suspected. The canals

are often equidistant from the midline and are connected by an isthmus. Occasionally, the main canal will bifurcate several millimetres below the pulp floor. Usually the point of confluence can be seen directly when using a microscope.

## Two Canals in Mandibular Incisors

A common reason for failure of root canal treatment in mandibular incisors occurs when a second canal has not been located and, consequently, is not disinfected. Approximately 41% of mandibular incisors will have two canals. The canals may be missed due to incorrect positioning of the access cavity. If access is too small or has been prepared too far lingually, it may be impossible to locate the lingual canal. To gain entry into a lingual canal, the access cavity may sometimes need to be extended very near to the incisal edge.

## Two Canals in a Mandibular Premolar

A lingual canal may be present in 11% of mandibular premolars. The canal normally projects from the wall of the main canal at an acute angle. It can usually be located by running a fine (ISO 08 or 10) file with a sharp bend in the tip along the lingual wall of the canal. Once an estimation of depth is made, the catch point may be visualized using the microscope. A small LN bur can be used to create a ledge at this point. Instruments will subsequently be guided into the orifice. A rotary nickel–titanium instrument such as a ProTaper SX (Maillefer, Ballaigues, Switzerland) can be used to funnel the orifice (Figure 6.31).

## *Bypassing Ledges*

Ledging occurs more frequently with filing techniques than balanced force instrumentation.[17,18] The latter technique utilizes non-end cutting, flexible files in a rotational motion. A filing action is rarely used in modern endodontics. Ledges can be created with Gates–Glidden burs during coronal flaring, but this can be avoided if the bur is used to

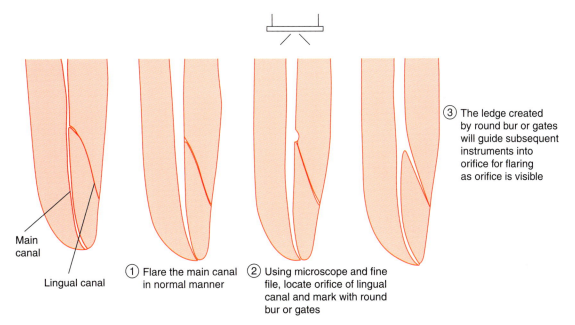

Main
canal

Lingual canal

① Flare the main canal
  in normal manner

② Using microscope and fine
  file, locate orifice of lingual
  canal and mark with round
  bur or gates

③ The ledge created
  by round bur or gates
  will guide subsequent
  instruments into
  orifice for flaring
  as orifice is visible

**Figure 6.31**

Negotiating the lingual canal in a mandibular premolar.

plane the wall of the root canal as it is withdrawn rather than being forced apically as if drilling down the root canal. Repeated recapitulation or remaining stationary in the canal with a non-landed rotary instrument can lead to apical transportation. Despite being very flexible, nickel–titanium instruments will impart a restoring force against the outer curvature of the canal. Files such as the ProTaper (Dentsply-Maillefer, Weybridge, Survey, UK) are highly efficient at machining dentine and the larger finishing files can, if misused, transport and ledge the canal.

Ledging often occurs directly following blockage of the canal with dentine chips. Inadequate irrigation, poor pilot channel preparation or recapitulation can lead to the packing of dentine chips and debris into the canal. When a rotary instrument hits the packed debris, it will either bind and separate or start transporting the canal, thereby forming a ledge.

To negotiate a ledge, the canal is flooded with EDTA gel and a precurved fine file introduced (ISO 8 or 10). The file is worked with a gentle watch-winding action to loosen any dentine chips at the point of blockage. When patency is regained, the instrument is worked up and down 1–2 mm a few times to ensure that a pilot channel is created. When the instrument is removed, the canal is irrigated with sodium hypochlorite to flush out any dentine chips (effervescence may possibly help in the process) (Figures 6.32, 6.33).

A persistent blockage may be fragmented using endosonics. The file should be used at low power with full irrigant flow to dislodge any dentine chips or material. Occasionally, using the operating microscope, a blockage may be visible and can be removed with a very fine ultrasonic tip such as the CPR 6, 7 or 8 or endosonics can be used. The tip of a size 15 endosonic file can be removed to create a more aggressive cutting instrument which will only need to be used on low power. The file tip can be bent to allow direct vision at the working site when using a microscope. A hand file can be modified in a similar manner to create a very efficient cutting instrument. It should not be used blind, however, since this is likely to result in transportation of the root canal (Figures 6.34–6.38).

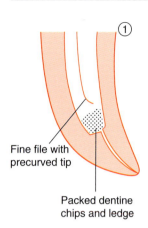
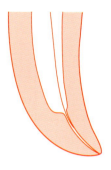
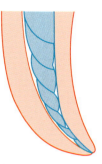

Fine file with
precurved tip

Packed dentine
chips and ledge

②  Place EDTA gel and
    pick and watch-wind with
    a fine file. Once root canal
    is engaged perform 4–5 filing
    motions to create pilot channel

③  The pilot channel can
    be engaged with a
    precurved nickel–titanium
    hand file. The tapered
    instrument will smooth
    the ledge

**Figure 6.32**

Negotiating a ledge.

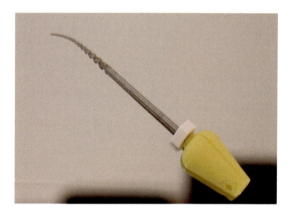

**Figure 6.33**

Once a ledge has been negotiated, a precurved nickel–
titanium hand instrument can be used to flare the root
canal beyond the ledge, thus reducing the step.

## Achieving Patency

Patency of the root canal can be lost if
dentine chips are compacted into the apical
part of the root canal system during preparation. This is more likely to occur if
insufficient irrigant is used during preparation. There are benefits in achieving patency
in infected root canals to ensure efficient

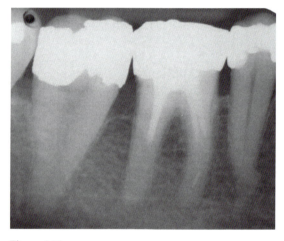

**Figure 6.34**

In this mandibular molar, ledges have been created
in the mesial root canals. The root canals are under-
prepared and the root filling material is short in both
mesial and distal roots. The gutta percha root filling was
easily removed with Gates–Glidden burs followed by
solvent. A fine precurved hand instrument was then
inserted and directed towards the midline area. The
mesial canals were renegotiated and could be refined
with nickel–titanium instruments. In the distal canal, a
previous attempt had ledged midway down the root.
Having removed material from the coronal aspect,
the root canal orifice could be visualized under the
operating microscope and was then prepared in the
normal manner.

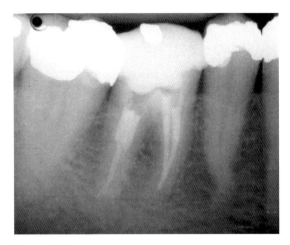

**Figure 6.35**

The case has been obturated with a vertically compacted gutta percha technique and the access cavity sealed ready for restoration with a Nayyar core.

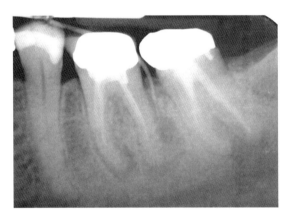

**Figure 6.36**

This mandibular molar has been poorly root filled. The canals are under-prepared, under-filled and the root filling material is short in both mesial and distal roots. There was a buccal sinus tract which could be delineated with a gutta percha cone. This traced to the distal root canal around which there was a large periapical radiolucency. The mesial canals were both ledged and required renegotiation. The gutta percha was removed using Gates–Glidden burs, Hedstroem files and chloroform. The root canals were then renegotiated, prepared and shaped using nickel–titanium rotary instruments.

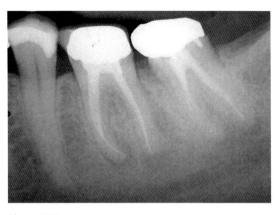

**Figure 6.37**

The case was irrigated with 4% sodium hypochlorite and EDTA and medicated with calcium hydroxide for 1 week prior to obturation with a vertically compacted gutta percha technique. The access cavity, which was made through an existing restoration, was sealed with IRM.

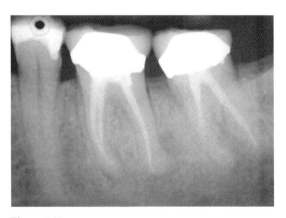

**Figure 6.38**

Six months following obturation, there was good evidence of bony healing.

distribution of irrigant into lateral canals and apical deltas. However, the benefit of patency has been questioned in cases where preventative retreatment is being carried out.[19,20] If there is no pathway for bacteria or their byproducts to exit the root canal, an inflammatory response will not be seen at the periapex. Patency filing in retreatment cases with no evidence of periapical disease may create an avenue for the supply of nutrients to bacteria within the root canal. Ironically, this could lead to the formation of a periapical area where one was not present prior to retreatment.

## REFERENCES

1. Fuss Z, Trope M. Root perforations: classification and treatment choices based on prognostic factors. *Endodontics and Dental Traumatology* 1996; **12**: 255–264.
2. Fridland M, Rosado R. Mineral trioxide aggregate (MTA) solubility and porosity with different water-to-powder ratios. *Journal of Endodontics* 2003; **29**: 814–817.
3. Torabinejad M, Watson TF, Pitt Ford TR. Sealing ability of mineral trioxide aggregate when used as a root end filling material. *Journal of Endodontics* 1993; **19**: 591–595.
4. Soluti A, Lee SJ, Torabinejad M. Sealing ability of mineral trioxide aggregate in lateral perforations. *Journal of Endodontics* 1993; **19**: 199.
5. Pitt Ford TR, Torabinejad M, McKendry DJ, Hong CU, Kariywasam SP. Use of mineral trioxide aggregate for repair of furcal perforations. *Oral Surgery, Oral Medicine, Oral Radiology and Endodontics* 1995; **79**: 756–762.
6. Holland R, de Souza V, Nery MJ, Otoboni Filho JA, Bernabe PF, Dezan E. Mineral trioxide aggregate repair of lateral root perforations. *Journal of Endodontics* 2001; **27**: 281–284.
7. Mitchell PJ, Pitt Ford TR, Torabinejad M, McDonald F. Osteoblast biocompatibility of mineral trioxide aggregate. *Biomaterials* 1999; **20**: 167–173.
8. Torabinejad M, Hilga RK, McKendry DJ, Pitt Ford TR. Dye leakage of four root end filling materials. Effects of blood contamination. *Journal of Endodontics* 1994; **20**: 159–163.
9. Oynick J, Oynick T. A study of a new material for retrograde fillings. *Journal of Endodontics* 1978; **4**: 203–206.
10. Dorn SO, Gartner AH. Retrograde filling materials: a retrospective success-failure study of amalgam, EBA and IRM. *Journal of Endodontics* 1990; **16**: 391–393.
11. Chong BS, Pitt Ford TR, Hudson M. A prospective study of Mineral Trioxide Aggregate and IRM when used as root-end filling materials in endodontic surgery. *International Endodontic Journal* 2003; **36**: 520–526.
12. Crooks WG, Anderson RW, Powell BJ, Kimbrough WF. Longitudinal evaluation of the seal of IRM root end fillings. *Journal of Endodontics* 1994; **20**: 250–252.
13. Lemon RR. Nonsurgical repair of perforation defects. Internal matrix concept. *Dental Clinics of North America* 1992; **36**: 439–457.
14. Bargholtz C. Perforation repair with mineral trioxide aggregate: a modified matrix concept. *International Endodontic Journal* 2005; **38**: 59–69.
15. Yoshioka T, Kobayashi C, Suda H. Detection rate of root canal orifices with a microscope. *Journal of Endodontics* 2002; **28**: 452–453.
16. von Arx T. Frequency and type of canal isthmuses in first molars detected by endoscopic inspection during periradicular surgery. *International Endodontic Journal* 2005; **38**: 160–168.
17. Sabala CL, Roane JB, Southard LZ. Instrumentation of curved canals using a modified tipped instrument: a comparison study. *Journal of Endodontics* 1988; **14**: 59–64.
18. Sepic AO, Pantera EA, Neaverth EJ, Anderson RW. A comparison of Flex-R file and K-type files for enlargement of severely curved molar root canals. *Journal of Endodontics* 1989; **15**: 240–245.
19. Bergenholtz G, Lekholm U, Milthon R, Heden G, Ödesjö B, Engström B. Retreatment of endodontic fillings. *Scandinavian Journal of Dental Research* 1979; **87**: 217–223.
20. Bergenholtz G, Lekholm U, Milthon R, Engström B. Influence of apical overinstrumentation and overfilling on re-treated root canals. *Journal of Endodontics* 1979; **5**: 310–314.

# 7 IRRIGATION AND MEDICATION

## INTRODUCTION

A large proportion of teeth that are root canal retreated are associated with intraradicular bacterial infection. As discussed in Chapter 1, this is an important factor that affects the outcome of endodontic treatment.[1,2] Available evidence shows that achieving adequate disinfection of the root canal system will increase the probability of success. Endodontic treatment employs an aseptic technique during which the infected root canal is disinfected using a combination of mechanical and chemical procedures.

The bacteria colonizing the root canal exist in a synergistic relationship and have evolved multiple nutritional interactions to survive in the nutrient-depleted conditions of the root canal. Primary endodontic treatment disrupts this environment. Some bacteria will be killed directly by chemomechanical preparation whilst others are killed indirectly by interfering with their nutritional supply. The importance of indirect killing should not be underestimated as this may be a means by which bacteria can be eradicated from the root canal in places where irrigants and medicaments have not been effective. Those that survive will be more hardy and resistant to treatment.

The root canal system is complex and includes many accessory anatomical features such as fins, lateral canals and intracanal communications.[3] In the infected root canal these voids are potential sites where bacterial colonization could take place. Some species of bacteria have also been identified in dentinal tubules. Invasion of tubules may extend 300 μm into the dentine of an infected tooth.[4] The ecosystem for bacterial colonization in the root-treated tooth differs from that of a primary infection. As bacteria all have specific ecological niches and nutritional interrelationships,[5] this environment may result in selected colonization by specific species. Commonly isolated microorganisms include cocci, rods, filamentous bacteria and fungi.[6] Microorganisms exist in planktonic form as a suspension within the root canal lumen and as complex coaggregates surrounded by amorphous material or plaque on the dentine wall of the root canal. The term 'biofilm' has been used to describe this feature of root canal infection.[7]

Studies utilizing culturing techniques have occasionally highlighted the presence of monoinfections in the root canals of endodontically treated teeth. However, this could well be a reflection of the method of analysis employed, since techniques using DNA, RNA and polymerase chain reaction (PCR) have demonstrated the presence of bacteria that are not cultivable. Bacteria such as *Enterococcus faecalis* and fungi such as *Candida albicans* have been isolated from root canals and have managed to survive endodontic cleaning and shaping.[8,9] These microorganisms have all been associated with the failure of root canal treatment. It will be interesting to see whether other non-cultivable resistant organisms are isolated in the future.

When bacteria have formed themselves into a complex biofilm, they often develop increased resistance to hostile external influences such as host defences, endodontic disinfectants, antibiotics and mechanical stress. Several hypotheses have been proposed to explain the mechanisms of biofilm resistance to antimicrobial agents:[10,11]

- bacterial exo-polysaccharide matrix may inactivate irrigants, preventing penetration into the biofilm

- bacterial cells undergo a stress response and enter a 'dormant' state during which metabolic processes are slowed and the bacteria are protected from antimicrobial agents
- bacterial expression of active mechanisms to combat the detrimental effects of antimicrobial agents.

As a result, established bacterial colonies within an infected root canal can be difficult to eradicate by chemical and mechanical means. The material properties of dentine can also reduce the antimicrobial activity of commonly used irrigating solutions and intracanal medicaments.[12]

A chemomechanical approach to disinfection of root canals has been adopted in modern endodontics. However the infected root canal may not always be sterilized using such a method.[1] Irrigating solutions are used during the preparation of root canals in order to attempt disinfection while the patient is in the surgery. There are many commonly used irrigants and others which may be used as adjuncts. For teeth with evidence of periapical pathology, a multiple-visit approach is often utilized and the prepared root canal space is completely occluded with a medicament between visits.

## IRRIGATING SOLUTIONS

Commonly used irrigants in endodontic treatment include:

- sodium hypochlorite
- iodine solutions
- chlorhexidine gluconate
- EDTA – ethylenediaminetetraacetic acid
- citric acid
- MTAD – mixture of tetracycline and disinfectant
- EAW – electrochemically activated water
- PAD – photoactivated disinfection
- ozone
- Endox.

Medicaments used in endodontic treatment include:

- calcium hydroxide
- iodine and iodine and calcium hydroxide mixtures
- antibiotics.

### Sodium Hypochlorite

Sodium hypochlorite has long been used in medicine as a safe antimicrobial agent. Buffered 0.5% sodium hypochlorite solution was used for wound cleaning during World War I.[13] The solution was shown to be an effective bactericidal agent without being toxic or interfering with healing.[14] Sodium hypochlorite was first introduced into endodontics by Gutheridge in 1919.[15] It is highly bactericidal and very effective at dissolving necrotic material. It has been advocated for use in endodontics in concentrations ranging from 0.5 to 5.25%, but there has been no agreement on the optimal concentration. Commercially available sodium hypochlorite, such as thin household bleach, would normally have a concentration of approximately $4 \pm 0.5\%$. The solutions are often very alkaline, hypertonic and highly irritant, and they may require dilution with 0.5% sodium bicarbonate before use as an endodontic irrigant. This will reduce the pH without affecting the bactericidal properties. Milton sterilizing fluid (Proctor & Gamble, Weybridge, Surrey, UK) is a stabilized 3% sodium hypochlorite solution and can be used as a root canal irrigant without dilution.

Although mechanical instrumentation and irrigation with copious amounts of sterile saline will reduce the number of bacteria in an infected root canal, a significantly greater reduction in the bacterial load can be achieved when using sodium hypochlorite solution as an irrigant.[16] No difference was found experimentally between a solution of 0.5 and 5.0%, but with lower concentrations the efficacy decreases rapidly, requiring copious irrigation to remain effective.[17] Sodium hypochlorite solution also deteriorates on storage and becomes less active with time, increased temperature, exposure to light or contamination with metallic ions.

With higher concentrations great care must be exercised by the operator to avoid extrusion into the periapical tissues,[18] because hypertonic and highly alkaline commercial bleach solutions are irritant and cytotoxic. When irrigating with sodium hypochlorite, it is advisable to use a small-bore safe-ended needle. The needle is marked with a rubber stop at the working length to prevent irrigant extrusion

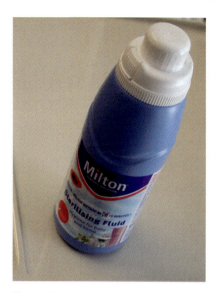

**Figure 7.1**

Milton solution is a 3% sodium hypochlorite solution stabilized with 16% sodium chloride.

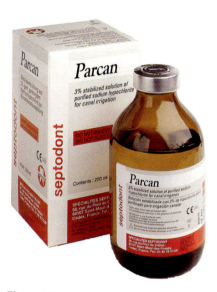

**Figure 7.2**

Parcan is a 3% stabilized solution of sodium hypochlorite.

and the tip of the needle is kept constantly in motion to prevent jamming in the root canal. A 1.0% sodium hypochlorite solution should be effective in removing root canal debris and dissolving organic matter and even at 0.5% solution is very potent at killing enterococci.[19] Work published by Baker et al using SEM analysis of root canals concluded that the volume of irrigant was more important than the type.[20] The volume of irrigant that can be contained in the root canal system is small and it can be rapidly inactivated. Regular replacement and agitation is required to maximize the effectiveness. Sodium hypochlorite has been shown to be effective for cleaning the apical part of root canals,[21] and in concentrations ranging from 1.0 to 6.0% it was effective in removing debris from the root canal (Figures 7.1–7.4).[22,23]

## Iodine Solutions

Iodine in potassium iodide solution has been recommended as a potential root canal irrigant because E. faecalis is sensitive to it. Safavi et al[24] showed that a 10-minute irrigant–dentine contact time on dentine infected with E. faecium was sufficient to prevent growth. In practice, a

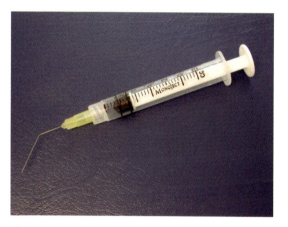

**Figure 7.3**

A 27-gauge monojet irrigating syringe. The needle has a safe-ended tip to prevent extrusion of irrigant.

solution of 5% iodine in potassium iodide or Churchill's solution can be used. Churchill's solution consists of iodine (16.5 g), potassium iodide (3.5 g), distilled water (20 g) and 90% ethanol (60 g). The presence of smear may decrease the effectiveness of the irrigant and it should therefore be used after smear removal.

In a study by Abdullah et al,[11] a strain of E. faecalis was isolated from an infected root canal associated with periapical disease and cultured as a planktonic suspension, a biofilm

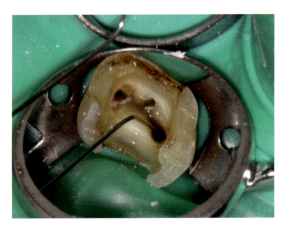

**Figure 7.4**

During irrigation of the root canal, the needle is kept constantly in motion. The plunger is depressed very slowly with a finger and the needle bent at a marked length to prevent extrusion of irrigant.

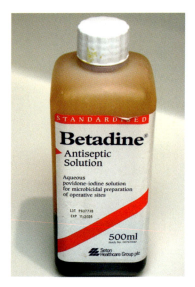

**Figure 7.5**

Betadine antiseptic solution is a povidone–iodine solution.

and a cell-dense pellet. Different irrigants and medicaments were then tested against the various presentations. A solution of 10% povidone–iodine (Betadine, Seton Healthcare, Oldham, UK) achieved a 100% bacterial kill in all samples of *E. faecalis* as a biofilm after exposure for both 2 and 30 minutes. The bacterial reductions for the planktonic presentation were higher than for the biofilm presentation, which in turn were higher than for the pellet presentation. These differences were significant ($p < 0.05$). Overall, povidone–iodine was not as effective as a 3% solution of sodium hypochlorite. Although the action of irrigant was considered to be affected by the anatomy and material properties of the dentine walls of a root canal, iodine solutions were considered to be a potentially useful adjunct to sodium hypochlorite, certainly for the killing of *E. faecalis*.

It is not uncommon to come across patients who are sensitive or allergic to iodine. Great care should be taken during history-taking to ascertain whether this is the case prior to using iodine-based irrigants and medicaments (Figure 7.5).

## Chlorhexidine Gluconate

The efficacy of chlorhexidine gluconate as an endodontic irrigant has recently been reinvestigated. It has a relatively broad spectrum of activity and low toxicity. Historically, it was not considered as a primary irrigant because of poor tissue-digesting properties. A 0.2% chlorhexidine gluconate solution (CHX) (Glaxo SmithKline Beecham, Brentford, Middlesex, UK) was tested against planktonic, biofilm and pellet presentations of *E. faecalis*. Although the solution showed the potential to reduce bacterial load, it was not as effective as 3% sodium hypochlorite or 10% povidone– iodine.[11] The bacterial reductions for the planktonic presentation were higher than for biofilm presentation, which in turn were higher than for the pellet presentation. These differences were significant ($p < 0.001$).

Chlorhexidine gluconate has good substantivity and has the ability to adhere to hydroxyapatite crystals in dentine. It has been postulated that it could potentially remain active following root canal treatment (Figure 7.6).[25]

## EDTA – Ethylenediaminetetraacetic acid

During root canal instrumentation, chips of dentine are removed from the root canal wall and a smear layer is produced. This is an amorphous, irregular, tenacious sludge and consists of organic and inorganic components such as odontoblast processes, microorganisms, pulp tissue and inorganic matrix from the dentine. Superficial smear is approximately 1–2 μm thick. However, it may be as thick as 40 μm in the deeper layers when material has been packed into dentine tubules. Smear can act as a reservoir for microorganisms. It could protect them from the action of antimicrobial irrigants when packed into dentinal tubules by preventing penetration of irrigants and medicaments. It may subsequently reduce the ability of sealers to penetrate the tubules during root canal obturation.

Although numerous studies have shown that sodium hypochlorite and saline solutions are ineffective at reducing smear layer, in areas where no smear has been formed sodium hypochlorite may remove predentine by a proteolytic effect.[22,23] Nygaard-Østby first introduced EDTA to endodontics as a means of softening dentine to make root canal preparation easier. Further research revealed that it was able to demineralize the root wall to a depth of approximately 20–50 μm particularly in the middle or coronal parts.[26] Chelating agents can be used to remove infected smear layer and open dentinal tubules, theoretically allowing more effective disinfection of the root canal system. The effectiveness of this protocol has yet to be scientifically proved in vivo,[17] but in-vitro removal of smear has been shown to aid irrigant penetration and bacterial killing.[27]

EDTA is also important for aiding biofilm removal. Its affinity for heavy metal ions causes the disruption of bacterial binding within the biofilm. EDTA is available in gel or aqueous form, usually in a concentration of 17% EDTA, and buffered to a neutral pH. Other chelating agents include 25% citric acid, 50% tannic acid and 40% polyacrylic acid. Chelating agents have direct and indirect antimicrobial actions. They may also be used as a lubricant to soften dentine and keep dentine chips in suspension.

The use of sodium hypochlorite or EDTA as a single irrigant will not remove all of the organic and inorganic debris. The rationale therefore has been to alternate these solutions in high volume.[23] It is interesting that using the solutions in the sequence EDTA, sodium hypochlorite and EDTA has proved to be more effective at removing smear layer than sodium hypochlorite, EDTA and sodium hypochlorite (Figures 7.7, 7.8).[28]

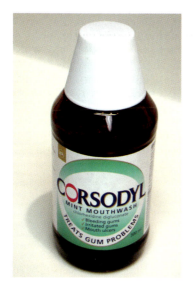

**Figure 7.6**

Corsodyl is a 0.2% chlorhexidine gluconate solution.

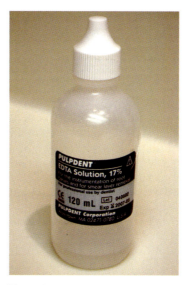

**Figure 7.7**

A 17% EDTA solution is normally used in endodontics. It is used to remove smear layer and can therefore be used in conjunction with other biologically active irrigants.

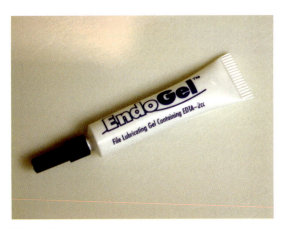

**Figure 7.8**

Lubricants used during mechanical preparation often contain EDTA. This helps prevent clogging of the root canal with dentine chips.

## Citric Acid

Citric acid has been used in endodontics as a chelating agent for some time.[29] It has been recommended as an irrigant in techniques such as photoactivated disinfection, where EDTA may have a detrimental effect on the action of the labelling agent.

## A Mixture of Tetracycline and Disinfectant

MTAD is a recently developed irrigating solution that consists of tetracycline, acetic acid and detergent.[30] Initial results show that MTAD may have some advantages over other irrigants and solutions used in root canal treatment. It will kill *E. faecalis*[31] and appears to be effective for removing smear layer along the entire length of the prepared root canal.[32] It is able to remove both organic and inorganic debris[33] but does not appear to have a detrimental effect on the physical dynamics of dentine, unlike 5.25% sodium hypochlorite and 17% EDTA. The MTAD solution may also be less cytotoxic than eugenol, 3% hydrogen peroxide, EDTA and calcium hydroxide.[34] The manufacturer's clinical protocol recommends

that MTAD should be used for 5 minutes as a final rinse after hypochlorite and EDTA. More independent research is required to evaluate the potential of this endodontic irrigant.

## Electrochemically Activated Water

When electrolysis of an aqueous saline solution is carried out in an EAW unit, an anolyte and a catholyte of electrochemically activated water are produced and isolated. The former is antimicrobial, has a high oxidation potential and pH of between 2 and 9.[35] When the anolyte and catholyte were individually used to irrigate infected canals, the antimicrobial effectiveness was disappointing when compared with 0.5% sodium hypochlorite.[36]

A newer solution, called electrolysed neutral water, produced a solution with a pH close to 7. This solution was bactericidal against a selection of commonly isolated endodontic pathogens.[37]

An alternative solution, termed oxidative potential water,[38] has been found to be highly antimicrobial because of its acidity and high oxidation–reduction potential. This solution has been shown to remove smear layer and debris when used to irrigate root canals.[39,40]

Sterilox (Optident, Peterborough, UK), is a commercially available unit that produces anolyte (Sterilox solution) and catholyte (sodium hydroxide pH 12.5) from a quality-controlled prepackaged solution. The main active ingredient that is produced by the Sterilox generator is 85–95% hypochlorous acid. This agent is a very effective biocide but is also non-toxic, non-sensitizing, non-irritating and non-mutagenic. The electrolyte is effective at removing the biofilm from dental water lines[41] and can be used as a surface disinfectant or for disinfecting impressions. It may be useful as an endodontic irrigant (Figures 7.9–7.10).

## Photoactivated Disinfection

The technique of photosensitization has been used in medicine for some time. PAD utilizes

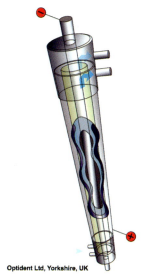

Optident Ltd, Yorkshire, UK

**Figure 7.9**

The Sterilox system utilizes a catalyst tube to produce two solutions from a quality-controlled prepackaged solution: Sterilox solution (anolyte) and sodium hydroxide (catholyte).

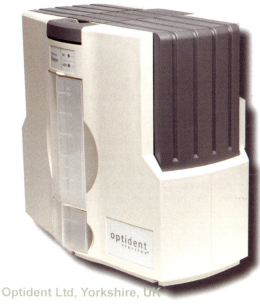

Optident Ltd, Yorkshire, UK

**Figure 7.10**

The Sterilox unit. Preprepared electrolyte is poured into the unit and the two solutions are then derived (Optident, Yorkshire, UK).

the photoactive agent tolonium chloride (toluidine chloride). The root canal is irrigated with the solution, which selectively binds to the cellular membrane of bacteria in the biofilm. The labelled bacterial cells rupture when exposed to laser light of the appropriate wavelength. The PAD system (Safedent: Denfotex Light Systems Ltd, Scotland, UK) uses a red laser-emitting radiation of wavelength 635 nm. The light is directed to the tip of a small flexible optical fibre that is inserted into the root canal. The maximum power setting of 100 mW ensures that the unit does not generate sufficient heat to harm the adjacent tissue. Tolonium chloride dye is biocompatible and will not stain dental tissue. Experimental data quoted by the manufacturer suggest that the PAD system has antimicrobial efficacies against commonly isolated oral bacteria.[42] In a paper by Seal et al, the PAD system was effective against *Streptococcus intermedius* biofilms in the root canal[43] but was not as effective as 3% sodium hypochlorite, which eliminated the entire bacterial population. Initial difficulties with the system arose because the laser light had not been transmitted correctly through the endodontic probe. The author commented that in infected root canals there may be complex anatomical features colonized by polymicrobial biofilms and, although sodium hypochlorite should still remain the primary irrigant of choice, PAD may be a useful adjunct. Early evidence from in-vivo experiments has shown that the PAD system appears to be effective in reducing bacterial load and helping achieve resolution of periapical periodontitis.[44,45]

Tolonium chloride, the labelling solution, is rendered ineffective by sodium hypochlorite and 3% EDTA. The manufacturers therefore recommend that the canal system is thoroughly washed out with sterile water, saline or citric acid before using it. Tolonium chloride is not proteolytic, and therefore irrigation with either sodium hypochlorite or citric acid is necessary. The dye is able to penetrate 100–150 μm into treated dentine and 60 μm without removal of smear. Increasing the contact time to over 4 minutes allows deeper penetration into the smear layer. The canal is irradiated for 150 seconds (Figures 7.11–7.13).

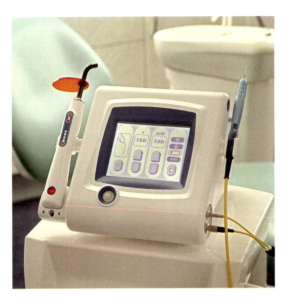

**Figure 7.11**

Photoactivated disinfection (PAD). The PAD system has an endodontic insert (on the right-hand side). This allows direction of red laser light into the root canal system (Denfotex, Scotland, UK).

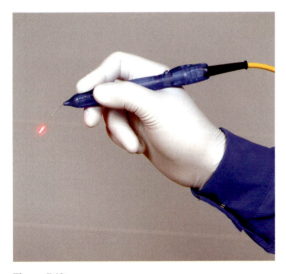

**Figure 7.12**

The PAD endotip (Denfotex, Scotland, UK).

## Ozone

Ozone is a powerful oxidizing agent and has high bactericidal properties. An ozone delivery unit has been manufactured for use in

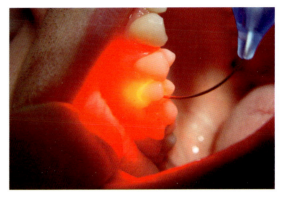

**Figure 7.13**

The PAD system being used to disinfect a disto-occlusal cavity in a premolar. The red laser light is visible, shining through the buccal aspect (Denfotex, Scotland, UK).

dentistry (HealOzone: CurOzone USA Inc, Farora, Canada). Initially, this device was used to reduce the microbial colonies associated with root caries. Attempts to sterilize the entire root canal system have proved complex, as perfusion of the gas is not reliable. In-vitro experiments have shown that ozone may be effective in killing planktonic *E. faecalis* but has little effect on *E. faecalis* embedded in biofilms.[46] Current recommendations from the Cochrane collaboration state that:

> Given the high risk of bias in the available studies and lack of consistency between different outcome measures, there is no reliable evidence that application of ozone gas to the surface of decayed teeth stops or reverses the decay process. There is a fundamental need for more evidence of appropriate rigour and quality before the use of ozone can be accepted into mainstream primary dental care or can be considered a viable alternative to current methods for the management and treatment of dental caries.[47]

There is some debate as to the antibacterial effectiveness, certainly in endodontics.

## Endox

The Endox Endodontic System (Lysis srl, Nova Milanese, Italy) has been reported to sterilize the root canal by emitting high-frequency electrical impulses. Sterilization occurs as a result of fulguration and the manufacturer claims it is able to eliminate both pulp and bacteria from the entire root canal system.[48] A recent study showed that the unit was not able to eliminate pulp tissue from the root canal system without mechanical cleaning. The authors could not recommend high-frequency electric pulses as the sole endodontic treatment but felt that the unit may be utilized as a supplement to traditional cleaning and shaping.[49]

## LASERS

There have been several drawbacks to the use of lasers in endodontics, including:

- the inability to deliver the laser light along a suitable fibre optic system
- the excessive heat generated by lasers, which may potentially damage periodontal tissue
- the cost
- the potential for genetic mutation when the wavelength of operation is close to the absorption peak of DNA.

Erbium lasers, which emit radiation at a wavelength similar to the absorption peak of water, have been considered suitable for the oblation of dentine, as they do not create too much heat.[50]

The Waterlase (Biolase, San Clemente, CA, USA) is an erbium–chromium–yttrium–scandium–gallium–garnet laser that has been claimed to exert hydrokinetic effects as the laser light reacts with water molecules. It has been reported that this laser is able to form the root canal shape without local anaesthesia.[51]

## DELIVERY OF IRRIGANTS

Root canal irrigants are normally introduced into the root canal system using a safe-ended endodontic syringe. Care must be taken to ensure that the needle tip does not bind, as irrigant may be forced through the apex. The tip can be premeasured and bent to avoid extrusion and the solution delivered slowly, without pressure.[52]

The root canal has to be prepared sufficiently for irrigant to penetrate the apical regions.[53,54] An ISO size 30 preparation appears to be adequate in most instances[55] to allow exchange. As discussed previously, the volume of solution appears to be a very important factor in achieving adequate disinfection. Inactivated irrigant needs to be constantly replenished.

It is harder to eliminate bacteria in biofilms than those in planktonic suspension. Mechanical agitation of the irrigant will help aid disruption of the multicellular biofilm structure. Ultrasonic irrigating devices have been suggested as a means of obtaining better irrigant delivery and mechanical agitation.[56] Agitation occurs by vibration of the file and acoustic microstreaming of the irrigant. Piezoelectric and magnetostrictive devices are both capable of delivering high volumes of irrigant, but the file tip may not vibrate if damped in highly curved or narrow canals,[57] and in this situation an alternative may be appropriate.

Recapitulation with a small file during preparation will help aid irrigant replenishment in the apical region and will also provide some mechanical agitation in areas where the instrument is able to contact the canal wall (Figure 7.14).

There are little published data regarding the optimal contact time for the various irrigants as most experimental work has been carried out *in vitro* and it is difficult to extrapolite this to the clinical situation. Subjective and anecdotal advice regarding the total irrigation time for root canal treatment has been placed at between 30–45 minutes.

### Culturing

Confirmation of a negative culture before obturating the root canal system has been shown to have a positive effect on treatment outcome and is a means of helping assess whether irrigants and medicaments have been successful in reducing or eliminating the bacterial load. Unfortunately, culturing is

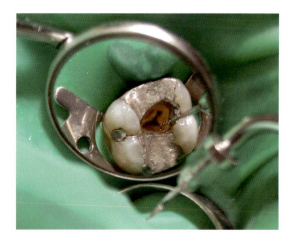

**Figure 7.14**

Endosonics being used to irrigate the root canal system of a maxillary molar.

extremely difficult in retreatment cases as many bacteria can be killed during removal of the existing root filling material. It is also apparent that bacteria which are inaccessible to irrigants and medicaments may prove elusive to sampling. Another major problem is the paucity of specialist microbiological centres available for the assessment of samples.

## MEDICAMENTS

Bacteria surviving preparation and irrigation will rapidly multiply between appointments if no intracanal medicament is used. Historically, vapour-forming agents such as formaldehydes and phenols were advocated: however, their duration of action and penetrating ability have been shown to be poor. They are carcinogenic and mutagenic[58] and can be distributed widely in the body. They have been shown to have only limited effectiveness[59] and, for this reason, there is little clinical evidence for using a phenol-based compound as an intracanal medicament.[60]

An inter-appointment medicament should be able to:

- continue the elimination of any bacteria remaining after chemomechanical preparation and long acting
- prevent coronal microleakage and not diffuse through the temporary restoration

- help dry a persistently wet canal
- not be inactivated by the presence of organic material, but should neutralize and dissolve any remaining tissue debris and degrade biofilm.
- decrease periapical inflammation and be of low toxicity to periapical tissues. It should not decrease the physical properties of the root structure.

The role of an intracanal medicament is secondary to the use of irrigant solution and should not be relied upon to provide disinfection of the root canal as a result of inadequate chemomechanical preparation.

### Calcium Hydroxide

Calcium hydroxide is a popular intracanal medicament[61] and has been used in dentistry since 1920. It has a good spectrum of antimicrobial activity and a long duration of action. It is relatively safe, easy to use and, in combination with sodium hypochlorite, may help dissolve retained organic material.[62] Calcium hydroxide is unfortunately not always effective at eliminating enterococci. These bacteria can be killed at pH 11.5, but attaining this level of alkalinity in the root canal is difficult.[12] *E. faecalis* uses a proton pump to control intracellular pH and this may be a means by which it can survive[63] high pH. During root canal retreatment, cultivable bacteria have been shown to survive despite two dressings with calcium hydroxide.[64] In fact, in this situation, the medicament may act as a selective medium for resistant bacteria. Some *Candida* species may also be resistant to calcium hydroxide. Calcium hydroxide is a slow-acting antibacterial agent and needs to be present in sufficient quantity and for at least 1 week in order to be effective.[65]

Commercially available preparations of calcium hydroxide vary in their presentation. In aqueous form calcium hydroxide is poorly dissociated but the hydroxyl ions liberated create the high pH that is required for bacterial killing. The majority of calcium hydroxide powder remains as a slurry in water, and this can result in poor flow characteristics. Dispersion into narrow or highly curved canals can be difficult. The slurry is thixotropic and with agitation becomes more fluid. It can therefore be

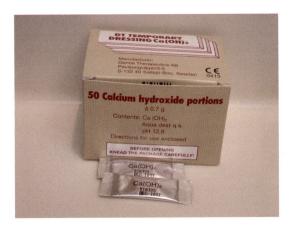

**Figure 7.15**

Sachets of 100% calcium hydroxide. The slurry can provide a pH of 12.6. This is sufficiently alkaline to kill most bacteria found in the root canal system but needs to be in contact with bacteria to be most effective.

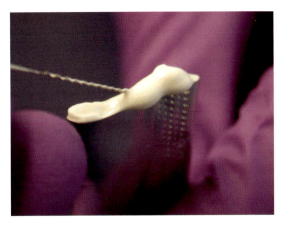

**Figure 7.17**

A lentulo spiral filler can be introduced into the sachet and will pick up calcium hydroxide. This can then be placed into the root canal.

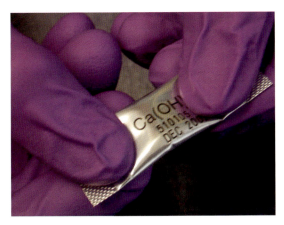

**Figure 7.16**

The calcium hydroxide sachet should be kneaded before use to thoroughly mix the contents.

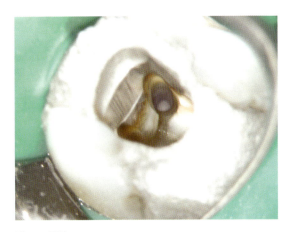

**Figure 7.18**

The mesiolingual root canal in this mandibular first molar has been fully prepared, irrigated and dried ready for the placement of calcium hydroxide medicament.

thick when dispensed but will flow when worked. The material can be introduced into the root canals with a Lentulo spiral filler or hand instrument. Calcium hydroxide can be mixed 7:1 with barium sulphate to make it radio-opaque. Some manufacturers mix the calcium hydroxide powder with glycerine, which improves flow but reduces pH and content of calcium hydroxide. Other carriers include methylcellulose, which also results in less disso-ciation. The carrier bases may make removal of the medicament more difficult.

Injectable calcium hydroxide pastes are available and are convenient to use, but ideally, single-use syringe tips should be employed to avoid cross-contamination. It is extremely difficult to sterilize syringe tips without risk of blockage (Figures 7.15–7.19).

### Iodine in Potassium Iodide

Antimicrobial agents such as iodine are pow-erful oxidizing agents that disrupt bacterial

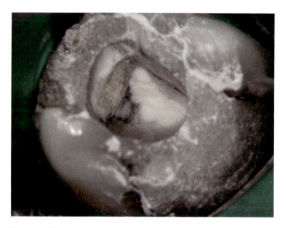

**Figure 7.19**

Calcium hydroxide has been spun into the root canal using a lentulo spiral filler, dried and packed into place.

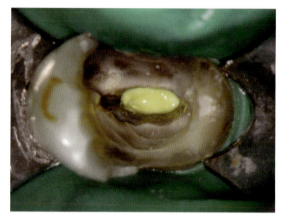

**Figure 7.21**

The calcium hydroxide and iodoform medicament (Metapex) has been placed in the root canal. The medicament is initially injected and then distributed using a hand file.

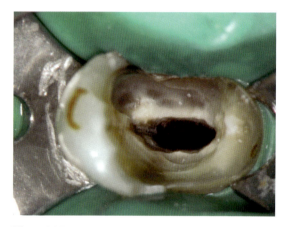

**Figure 7.20**

The root canal system in this premolar has been retreated and thoroughly disinfected. The canal has been dried ready for the placement of calcium hydroxide and iodoform medicament.

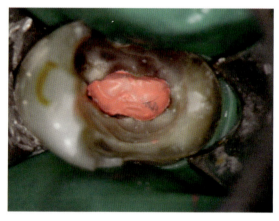

**Figure 7.22**

The coronal aspect is first sealed with a plug of thermoplasticized gutta percha and then the coronal aspect sealed with a resin-modified glass ionomer.

cellular enzyme systems and inactivate them. Iodine in potassium iodide (IPI) has been used in endodontics as an intracanal antiseptic agent in concentrations between 2 and 10% in aqueous solution. It is an effective antimicrobial with a broad spectrum and comparatively low toxicity.[24,66] The effectiveness of the solution is short-lived and is not suitable for periods of medication longer than 2 days. An alternative is to use IPI as an irrigant following smear removal and then place a mixture of IPI and calcium hydroxide as a medicament.[67]

Commercially available preparations of iodoform and calcium hydroxide, such as Metapex, are available. The material is highly radio-opaque and can be useful to confirm that the entire root canal system has been obliterated with medicament prior to sealing the access cavity (Figures 7.20–7.22).

## Antibiotics

Historically, pastes such as Grossman's polyantibiotic paste have been used as a medicament in root canal treatment. The paste contained penicillin, but, as most of the bacterial species found in the root canal are resistant due to their ability to produce the enzyme beta-lactamase, it is relatively ineffective.

Metronidazole is effective against Gram-negative anaerobes and has been used as an adjunct in periodontal treatment. It has been advocated for use as a root canal irrigant.[68] Tetracyclines have been used with some success in periodontal treatment. Doxycycline combined with corticosteroids are ingredients of Ledermix (Blackwell Supplies, Gillingham, Kent, UK). Unfortunately, the range and duration of antimicrobial action may be limited in the endodontic environment.[69,70] In addition, not all the constituents may be easily removed from the root canal prior to obturation, which could subsequently affect the quality of seal with gutta percha and sealer.[71] Mixing Ledermix with calcium hydroxide does not produce any synergistic effect and the two materials should not be used in combination.[72]

Clindamycin placed in teeth with necrotic pulps undergoing root canal treatment offered no advantage over conventional root canal dressings such as calcium hydroxide for elimination of bacteria. Its clinical use was not recommended.[73]

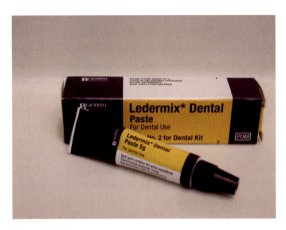

**Figure 7.23**

Ledermix paste. The use of an antibiotic paste as a root canal dressing is no more effective than calcium hydroxide. However, Ledermix can be a useful material for the emergency treatment of irreversible pulpitis.

There is the risk that without bacterial culturing or analysis, the injudicious use of antibiotics may result in bacterial resistance. An infected root canal contains a complex mixed flora and it is, therefore, inappropriate to rely on them to eliminate all of the bacteria.[74] Topical application of antibiotic may also increase the risk of a patient becoming sensitized to it (Figure 7.23).

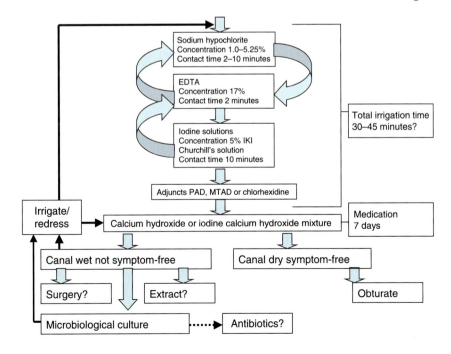

**Figure 7.24**

Irrigation and medication protocols for root canal retreatment. For abbreviations, please refer to the text.

## SINGLE-VISIT TREATMENT

Teeth that require root canal retreatment are very likely to be associated with bacterial infection. The time taken to isolate a tooth, dismantle previous restorations and root filling materials, identify and negotiate the canal system and then complete chemomechanical disinfection is much longer than that required for primary treatment. To what extent can all the steps required for quality retreatment be undertaken in a single visit? In a vital case or non-vital traumatic case there is a good argument for single-visit treatment, but in retreatment a multiple-visit strategy is normally adopted.[75]

Although some reports have shown that medicaments such as calcium hydroxide do not always render the root canal system bacteria-free, none has claimed that medicaments are totally ineffective at further reduction of the bacterial load following preparation and irrigation.

By adopting a two- or three-visit strategy, the clinician can monitor the resolution of pre-treatment signs and symptoms prior to obturation. If further disinfection is required or a flare-up occurs, it is much easier to access the root canal system.

## REFERENCES

1. Sjögren U, Figdor D, Persson S, Sundqvist G. Influence of infection at the time of root filling on the outcome of endodontic treatment of teeth with apical periodontitis. *International Endodontic Journal* 1997; **30:** 297–306.
2. Engström B. The significance of enterococci in root canal treatment. *Odontological Reviews* 1964; **15:** 87–105.
3. Vetucci FJ. Root canal anatomy of human permanent teeth. *Oral Surgery, Oral Medicine, Oral Pathology* 1984; **58:** 589–599.
4. Shovelton DS. The presence and distribution of microorganisms within non-vital teeth. *British Dental Journal* 1964; **117:** 101–107.
5. Pinheiro ET, Gomes BPFA, Ferraz CCR. Microorganisms from canals of root-filled teeth with periapical lesions. *International Endodontic Journal* 2003; **36:** 1–11.
6. Nair PN. Light and electron microscopic studies of root canal flora and periapical lesions. *Journal of Endodontics* 1987; **13:** 29–39.
7. Costerton JW, Geesey GG, Cheng KJ. How bacteria stick. *Scientific American* 1978; **238:** 86–95.
8. Waltimo TM, Sirén EK, Torkko HL, Olsen I, Haapasalo MP. Fungi in therapy-resistant apical periodontitis. *International Endodontic Journal* 1997; **30:** 96–101.
9. Molander A, Reit C, Dahlén G, Kvist T. Microbiological status of root-filled teeth with apical periodontitis. *International Endodontic Journal* 1998; **31:** 1–7.
10. Stewart PS, Costerton JW. Antibiotic resistance of bacteria in biofilms. *Lancet* 2001; **358:** 135–138.
11. Abdullah M, Ng YL, Gulabivala K, Moles DR, Spratt DA. Susceptibilties of two *Enterococcus faecalis* phenotypes to root canal medications. *Journal of Endodontics* 2005; **31:** 30–36.
12. Haapasalo HK, Sirén EK, Waltimo TM, Ørstavik D, Haapasalo MP. Inactivation of local root canal medicants by dentine: an in vitro study. *International Endodontic Journal* 2000; **33:** 126–131.
13. Dakin HD. The antiseptic action of hypochlorite. *British Medical Journal* 1915; **December:** 809–810.
14. Dakin HD. On the use of certain antiseptic substances in the treatment of infected wounds. *British Medical Journal* 1915; **August:** 327–331.
15. Coolidge E. The diagnosis and treatment of conditions resulting from diseased dental pulps. *Journal of the National Dental Association* 1919; **6:** 337–349.
16. Byström A, Sundqvist G. Bacteriologic evaluation of the effect of 0.5% sodium hypochlorite in endodontic therapy. *Oral Surgery, Oral Medicine, Oral Pathology* 1983; **55:** 307–312.
17. Byström A, Sundqvist G. The antibacterial effect of sodium hypochlorite and EDTA in 60 cases of endodontic therapy. *International Endodontic Journal* 1985; **18:** 35–40.
18. Becking AG. Complications in the use of sodium hypochlorite during endodontic

treatment. *Oral Surgery, Oral Medicine, Oral Pathology* 1991; **71**: 346–348.

19. Evans M, Davies JK, Sundqvist G, Figdor D. Mechanisms involved in the resistance of *Enterococcus faecalis* to calcium hydroxide. *International Endodontic Journal* 2002; **25**: 221–228.

20. Baker NA, Eleazer PD, Averbach RE, Seltzer S. Scanning electron microscopic study of the efficacy of various irrigating solutions. *Journal of Endodontics* 1975; **1**: 127–135.

21. Baumgartner JC, Brown CM, Mader CL, Peters DD, Shulman JD. A scanning electron microscope evaluation of root canal debridement using saline, sodium hypochlorite, and citric acid. *Journal of Endodontics* 1984; **11**: 525–531.

22. Baumgartner JC, Cuenin PR. Efficacy of several concentrations of sodium hypochlorite for root canal irrigation. *Journal of Endodontics* 1992; **18**: 605–612.

23. Baumgartner JC, Mader CL. A scanning electron microscope evaluation of four root canal irrigation regimes. *Journal of Endodontics* 1987; **13**: 147–157.

24. Safavi E, Spangberg L, Langeland K. Root canal dentine tubule disinfection. *Journal of Endodontics* 1990; **16**: 207–210.

25. Spangberg LSW, Haapasalo M. Rationale and efficacy of root canal medicaments and root filling materials with emphasis on treatment outcome. *Endodontic Topics* 2002; **2**: 35–58.

26. Fraser JG. Chelating agents: their softening effect on root canal dentine. *Oral Surgery, Oral Medicine, Oral Pathology* 1975; **37**: 803–836.

27. Ørstavik D, Haapasalo M. Disinfection by endodontic irrigants and dressings of experimentally infected dentine tubules. *Endodontics and Dental Traumatology* 1990; **6**: 142–149.

28 Abbott PV, Heijkoop PS, Cardaci SC, Hume WR, Heithersay GS. An SEM study of the effects of different irrigation sequences and ultrasonics. *International Endodontic Journal* 1991; **24**: 308–316.

29. Von der Fehr FR, Nygaard-Østby B. Effects of EDTAC and sulfuric acid on root canal dentine. *Oral Surgery, Oral Medicine, Oral Pathology* 1963; **16**: 199–205.

30. Torabinejad M, Khademi AA, Babogoli J. A new solution for the removal of smear layer. *Journal of Endodontics* 2003; **29**: 170–175.

31. Shabahang S, Torabinejad M. Effect of MTAD on *Enterococcus faecalis* contaminated root canals of extracted human teeth. *Journal of Endodontics* 2003; **29**: 576–579.

32. Torabinejad M, Cho Y, Khademi AA, Bakland LK, Shabahang S. The effect of various concentrations of sodium hypochlorite on the ability of MTAD to remove smear layer. *Journal of Endodontics* 2003; **29**: 233–239.

33. Beltz RE, Torabinejad M, Pouresmail M. Quantitative analysis of the solubilizing action of MTAD, sodium hypochlorite, and EDTA on bovine pulp and dentine. *Journal of Endodontics* 2003; **29**: 334–337.

34. Zhang W, Torabinejad M, Li Y. Evaluation of cytotoxicity of MTAD using the MTT-tetrazolium method. *Journal of Endodontics* 2003; **29**: 654–657.

35. Marais JT. Cleaning efficacy of a new root canal irrigation solution: a preliminary investigation. *International Endodontic Journal* 2000; **33**: 320–325.

36. Marais JT, Williams WP. Antimicrobial effectiveness of electrochemically activated water as an endodontic irrigation solution. *International Endodontic Journal* 2001; **34**: 237–243.

37. Horiba N, Hiratsuka K, Onoe T. Bactericidal effect of electrolyzed neutral water on bacteria isolated from infected root canals. *Oral Surgery, Oral Medicine, Oral Pathology, Oral Radiology and Endodontics* 1999; **87**: 83–87.

38. Hata G, Uemura S, Weine FS, Toda T. Removal of smear layer in the root canal using oxidative potential water. *Journal of Endodontics* 1996; **22**: 643–645.

39. Hata G, Hayami S, Weine FS, Toda T. Effectiveness of oxidative potential water as a root canal irrigant. *International Endodontic Journal* 2001; **34**: 308–317.

40. Solovyeva AM, Dummer PM. Cleaning effectiveness of root canal irrigation with electrochemically activated anolyte and catholyte solutions: a pilot study. *International Endodontic Journal* 2000; **33**: 494–504.

41. Marais JT, Brozel VS. Electro-chemically activated water in dental unit water lines. *British Dental Journal* 1999; **187:** 154–158.

42. Wilson M, Burns T, Pratten J, Pearson GJ. Bacteria in supra-gingival plaque samples can be killed by lower power laser light in the presence of photo-sensitiser. *Journal of Applied Bacteriology* 1995; **78:** 569–574.

43. Seal GJ, Ng YL, Spratt D, Bhatti M, Gulabivala K. An in vitro comparison of the bactericidal efficacy of lethal photo-sensitization or sodium hypochlorite irrigation on *Streptococcus intermedius* biofilms in root canals. *International Endodontic Journal* 2002; **35:** 268–274.

44. Bonsor SJ, Nichol R, Reid TMS, Pearson GJ. Microbiological evaluation of photo-activated disinfection in endodontics (an *in vivo* study). 2005; in press.

45. Bonsor SJ, Nichol R, Reid TMS, Pearson GJ. Alternative regimens for root canal irrigation. 2005; in press.

46. Hems RS, Gulabivala K, Ng Y, Ready D, Spratt DA. An in vitro evaluation of the ability of ozone to kill a strain of *Enterococcus faecalis. International Endodontic Journal* 2005; **38:** 22–29.

47. Rickard GD, Richardson R, Johnson T, McColl D, Hooper L. Ozone therapy for the treatment of dental caries. *The Cochrane Database of Systematic Reviews* 2004; Issue 3: www.update-software.com/Abstracts.

48. Endox Endodontic System: http://www.endox.com

49. Lendini M, Alemanno E, Migliaretti G, Beratti E. The effect of high-frequency electrical pulses on organic tissue in root canals. *International Endodontic Journal* 2005; **38:** 531–538.

50. Khabbaz MG, Makropoulou MI, Serafetinides AA, Papadopoulous D, Papagiakoumou E. Q-switched versus free-running Er-YAG laser efficacy on the root canal walls of human teeth: a SEM study. *Journal of Endodontics* 2004; **30:** 585–588.

51. Chen WH. YSGG laser root canal therapy. *Dentistry Today* 2002; **21:** 74–77.

52. Pitt Ford TR, Rhodes JS, Pitt Ford HE. *Endodontics: Problem solving in clinical practice.* London: Martin Dunitz; 2002.

53. Ram Z. Effectiveness of root canal irrigation. *Oral Surgery, Oral Medicine, Oral Pathology* 1977; **44:** 306–312.

54. Abou-Rass M, Piccinino MV. The effectiveness of four clinical irrigation methods on the removal of root canal debris. *Oral Surgery, Oral Medicine, Oral Pathology* 1982; **54:** 323–328.

55. Salzgeber RM, Brilliant JD. An in vivo evaluation of the penetration of an irrigating solution in root canals. *Journal of Endodontics* 1977; **3:** 394–398.

56. Cunningham WT, Martin H, Forrest WR. Evaluation of root canal debridement by the endosonic ultrasonic synergistic system. *Oral Surgery, Oral Medicine, Oral Pathology* 1982; **53:** 401–404.

57. Cheung GSP, Stock CJR. In vitro cleaning ability of root canal irrigants with and without endosonics. *International Endodontic Journal* 1993; **26:** 334–343.

58. Lewis BB, Chestner SB. Formaldehyde in dentistry: a review of mutagenic and carcinogenic potential. *Journal of the American Dental Association* 1981; **103:** 429–434.

59. Byström A, Claesson R, Sundqvist G. The antibacterial effect of camphorated para-monochlorophenol, camphorated phenol and calcium hydroxide in the treatment of infected root canals. *Endodontics and Dental Traumatology* 1985; **1:** 170–175.

60. Sipes R, Binkley CJ. The use of formocresol in dentistry: a review of the literature. *Quintessence International* 1986; **17:** 415–417.

61. Sjögren U, Figdor D, Spangberg L, Sundqvist G. The antimicrobial effect of calcium hydroxide as a short-term intra-canal dressing. *International Endodontic Journal* 1991; **24:** 119–125.

62. Hasselgren G, Olsson B, Cvek M. Effects of calcium hydroxide and sodium hypochlorite on the dissolution of necrotic porcine muscle tissue. *Journal of Endodontics* 1998; **14:** 125–127.

63. Evans M, Davies JK, Sundqvist G, Figdor D. Mechanisms involved in the resistance of *Enterococcus faecalis* to calcium hydroxide. *International Endodontic Journal* 2002; **35:** 221–228.

64. Sundqvist G, Figdor D, Persson S, Sjögren U. Microbiologic analysis of teeth with

failed endodontic treatment and the outcome of conservative retreatment. *Oral Surgery, Oral Medicine, Oral Pathology and Endodontics* 1998; **85:** 86–93.

65. Sjögren U, Figdor D, Spangberg L, Sundqvist G. The antimicrobial effect of calcium hydroxide as a short-term intracanal dressing. *International Endodontic Journal* 1991; **24:** 119–125.

66. Spangberg L, Engström B, Langeland K. Biological effect of dental materials. 3. Toxicity and antimicrobial effects of endodontic antiseptics in vitro. *Oral Surgery, Oral Medicine, Oral Pathology* 1973; **36:** 856–871.

67. Molander A, Reit C, Dahlen G, Kvist T. Microbiological status of root-filled teeth with apical periodontitis. *International Endodontic Journal* 1998; **31:** 1–7.

68. Sanjiwan R, Chandra S, Jaiswal JN, Mats AN. The effect of metronidazole on the anaerobic microorganisms of the root canal – a clinical study. *Federation of Operative Dentistry* 1990; **1:** 30–36.

69. Abbott PV, Heithersay GS, Hume WR. Release and diffusion through human tooth roots in vitro of corticosteroid and tetracycline trace molecules from Ledermix paste. *Endodontics and Dental Traumatology* 1988; **4:** 55–62.

70. Abbott PV, Hume WR, Pearman JW. Antibiotics and endodontics. *Australian Dental Journal* 1990; **35:** 50–60.

71. Harris BM, Wendt SL. The effects of a petroleum-based ointment and water-based cream on apical seal. *Journal of Endodontics* 1987; **13:** 122–125.

72. Seow WK. The effects of didactic combinations of endodontic medicaments on microbial growth inhibition. *Paediatric Dentistry* 1990; **12:** 292–297.

73. Molander A, Reit C, Dahlen G. Microbiological evaluation of clindamycin as a root canal dressing in teeth with apical periodontitis. *International Endodontic Journal* 1990; **23:** 113–118.

74. Chong BS, Pitt Ford TR. The role of intracanal medication in root canal treatment. *International Endodontic Journal* 1992; **25:** 97–106.

75. Sjögren U, Hagglund B, Sundqvist G, Wing K. Factors affecting the long-term results of endodontic treatment. *Journal of Endodontics* 1990; **16:** 498–504.

# 8 INTRODUCTION TO SURGICAL ENDODONTICS

**CONTENTS • Introduction • Prognosis for Endodontic Surgery • Current Indications for Surgery • Contraindications to Surgical Endodontics • Preoperative Planning • References**

## INTRODUCTION

The main aim of root canal treatment is to clean and disinfect the root canal system, thereby reducing the bacterial load, removing necrotic tissue and creating an environment in which periapical healing can occur. Non-surgical retreatment is considered to provide a better opportunity to disinfect the root canal system than a surgical approach, as it is generally not possible to clean the coronal part of the root canal system during endodontic surgery.[1]

## PROGNOSIS FOR ENDODONTIC SURGERY

Many studies have been published on the prognosis of endodontic surgery but, as with non-surgical retreatment, there is considerable variation in the methods that have been utilized. The approach described by Molven et al[2] has been universally accepted and shows good correlation with histological assessment.[3] The outcome following endodontic surgery is classified by four categories:

- complete healing
- incomplete healing (scar)
- uncertain healing
- failure.

Long-term follow-up may be required to ascertain the outcome for cases showing uncertain healing, as there can be both late success and failure. Review earlier than 1 year is generally inconclusive, and follow-up is recommended for at least 4 years.[4] As with primary treatment and retreatment, the presence of periapical pathology and an infected root canal, or poor root treatment, will have a negative effect on the prognosis of surgical treatment.[5–9] Most surgical failures are the result of poor disinfection of the root canal[10] and, consequently, it is usually preferable to have completed non-surgical retreatment prior to endodontic surgery (Figures 8.1, 8.2).

There are situations in which a non-surgical approach may not be feasible, but since the introduction of operating microscopes in endodontics there are now probably fewer indications for using a surgical approach.[11,12] The techniques available to the endodontist using a conventional approach have improved enormously and the predictability of dismantling root fillings to enable disinfection of the root canal system has increased.

## CURRENT INDICATIONS FOR SURGERY

1. When conventional treatment or retreatment has failed. Surgical endodontics may be considered in a root-filled tooth with the presence of periradicular disease (with or without symptoms) when non-surgical root canal retreatment cannot be undertaken or has failed or where conventional retreatment may be detrimental to the retention of the tooth (Figures 8.3–8.6).[12]

2. When root canal treatment or retreatment is impractical or there is a strong possibility of

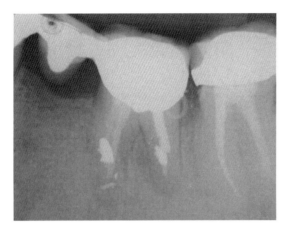

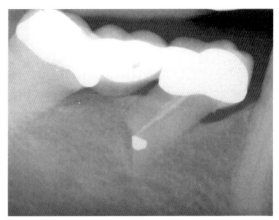

**Figure 8.1**

Root end surgery has been carried out on this mandibular molar, which is the distal abutment of a fixed bridge. The root ends have been severely bevelled and the canals inadequately prepared. The amalgam retrograde fillings do not provide an adequate seal. The mesiolingual canal appears not to have been prepared and bacterial irritants from both mesial and distal root canals will be leaking past the retrograde fillings. Root end resection has resulted in significant shortening of both roots. The distal root has fractured and unfortunately the tooth is now unsaveable. Non-surgical root canal treatment could probably have been attempted and the presence of a post is no longer an indication for root end surgery.

**Figure 8.2**

Root end resection and filling with amalgam has been carried out on this mandibular premolar. The bevel is excessive, which has significantly shortened the root. This may have been the result of difficult access. The root canal has not been prepared and the amalgam root end filling is not providing a seal. Unfortunately, this case has now been severely compromised. The root filling is technically deficient and there is evidence of periapical radiolucency. A non-surgical approach would probably have been more appropriate.

failure. Surgery may be required when iatrogenic events, pathological processes or developmental anomalies prevent a non-surgical approach in a tooth with periradicular pathology.

3. When biopsy or investigation is required. Sometimes a biopsy of periradicular tissue is required or direct visualization of the periradicular tissues and tooth root is needed in order to assess a perforation or to confirm the presence of root fracture or cracking. Foreign material that has been extruded from the root canal and appears to be associated with an inflammatory reaction or infection should be removed (Figures 8.7–8.9).[13,14]

4. As a combined approach with a non-surgical technique. Surgery will be used in combination with non-surgical treatment if tooth sectioning or root amputation is required. This may be as a result of periodontal and endodontic disease (Figure 8.10).

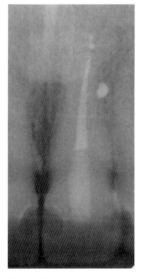

**Figure 8.3**

The root canal treatment in this maxillary incisor has a good radiographic appearance. The tooth was still symptomatic several months after obturation and there was tenderness over the apex. Non-surgical retreatment would be the first line of treatment.

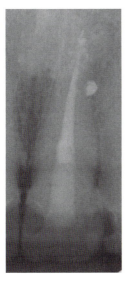

**Figure 8.4**

Root canal retreatment has been completed and as a result of further irrigation an apical delta has been revealed following obturation. It was not possible to remove the extruded gutta percha from a lateral canal in the mid-third. Unfortunately, despite a thorough approach to root canal retreatment, the tooth was still symptomatic. Root end surgery was therefore indicated.

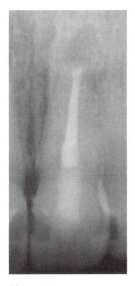

**Figure 8.5**

The maxillary incisor following root resection, preparation and placement of an MTA root end filling. Extruded gutta percha has been removed from the lateral canal and the gutta percha burnished. The tooth was symptom-free following surgery.

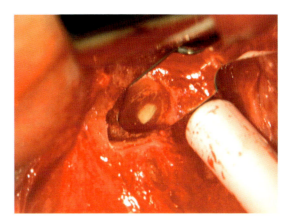

**Figure 8.6**

Inspection of the MTA root end filling prior to flap closure.

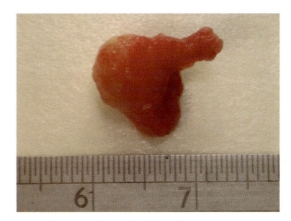

**Figure 8.7**

A biopsy can be required when a suspicious lesion is present at the periapex. An indication of size should be recorded and the sample sent in formal saline to a histopathology laboratory for assessment. In this case a lesion has been curetted in toto.

5. Where it may not be expedient to undertake prolonged surgical root canal retreatment because of patient factors.[11]

## CONTRAINDICATIONS TO SURGICAL ENDODONTICS

Most endodontic surgery is generally carried out using local analgesia and there are

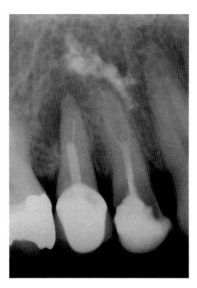

**Figure 8.8**

In this case a significant amount of paste has been extruded from the maxillary first premolar. There is evidence of radiolucency around the material. As the root filling in this premolar was inadequate, a combined approach to treatment was recommended. The tooth was first treated using a non-surgical approach to ensure that the root canals were adequately cleaned and filled. A surgical approach was used to remove extruded material. At the same time, the second premolar was treated using a surgical approach, as it was felt that dismantling the restoration may result in the tooth becoming non-viable.

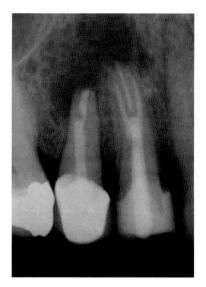

**Figure 8.9**

Root end surgery has been completed on the maxillary premolars. The first premolar was retreated using a non-surgical approach. During surgery, extruded material was removed from the bone surrounding the root apices and the root ends resected. It was felt that root end filling was not necessary in this case as root canal retreatment had only recently been completed. The gutta percha was therefore burnished. In the second premolar, the root end was resected and a separated instrument retrieved from the root canal. This was then prepared using ultrasonic tips and sealed with MTA.

relatively few contraindications. However, a comprehensive medical history should be taken and patient consent obtained prior to treatment. Psychological considerations and the presence of severe systemic disease may preclude the use of surgery. Anatomical factors, including unusual bone or root configurations, poor surgical access, possible involvement of neurovascular tissue or poor supporting tissues, may prevent surgical treatment. The skill, training and expertise of the operator will have an influence on the suitability of using a surgical approach and referral to a specialist colleague may be appropriate.

## PREOPERATIVE PLANNING

Factors that should be considered during surgical planning include those relating to the patient, the anatomy and the clinician. Practitioners accepting referrals are more likely to be treating difficult cases and patients with complex medical problems.

### Patient Factors

#### Psychological Factors and Assessment of Patient Cooperation

Patients who are dental phobic or perhaps very anxious about dental treatment may require counselling before starting treatment and could benefit from conscious sedation.

#### Systemic Disease

Although there are few general systemic contraindications for endodontic surgery, it

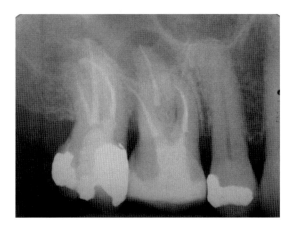

**Figure 8.10**

The maxillary first molar has a large periodontal defect associated with it. As part of an overall treatment plan, it was intended to resect this root. Endodontic treatment has been completed in a conventional manner and the coronal part of the root canal filled with composite. Resection of the root can be carried out surgically.

may be necessary to liaise with a patient's specialist in order to assess their suitability for surgical treatment under local anaesthetic. Factors may become more complex if general anaesthesia is to be considered. Such systemic conditions could include the following conditions.

*Cardiac Disease*
Severe hypertension can increase the risk of operative complications and postoperative bleeding. If the blood pressure is significantly raised, treatment should be postponed until this is brought under control by a medical specialist.[15] Drugs such as beta-blockers and non-potassium-sparing diuretics can exacerbate the unwanted effects of adrenaline (epinephrine) in dental local anaesthetics, and dose reduction should be considered. Patients with cardiac arrhythmias and those who have had cardiac transplantation are sensitive to adrenaline- containing local anaesthetics, which should be avoided.[16] Patients who are medicated for angina should have their medication available should it be required. Sedation should be used with caution, as it may mask symptoms of angina. In patients who have suffered myocardial infarction, elective surgery

should be postponed for at least 3 months and, ideally, 1 year. A previous history of infective endocarditis, rheumatic fever or heart valve disease or surgery will require antibiotic prophylaxis.

*Respiratory Disease*
Patients with chronic obstructive airways disease (COAD) such as chronic bronchitis and emphysema can have difficulty lying supine for long periods.[17] The use of a rubber dam may not be possible without low-concentration, supplemental oxygen via a nasal cannula. In cases of severe asthma or emphysema, intravenous sedation should be avoided due to the risk of respiratory depression. Patients should be encouraged to use their salbutamol inhaler prior to the commencement of surgery.[15]

*Haematological Disorders*
Surgery for patients undergoing treatment for leukaemia should be performed during stages of remission and between chemotherapeutic regimens. The specialist haematologist should be consulted. Patients with congenital bleeding disorders such as haemophilia A, Christmas disease or von Willebrand's disease should be treated in a specialist centre. Inferior alveolar nerve blocks are contraindicated in patients with bleeding disorders unless suitable prophylaxis has been provided, as a bleed may track around the pharynx, leading to airway obstruction.[18]

*Endocrine Disorders*
Diabetics should be the first to be treated in the morning having eaten prior to surgery.[15] Patients taking oral hypoglycaemics should omit the morning dose of oral hypoglycaemic and recommence therapy postoperatively. The patient should be monitored for signs of hypoglycaemia. All diabetics are at an increased risk of postoperative infection and should be prescribed appropriate antibiotics. Erythromycin may interact with glibenclamide and precipitate hypoglycaemia.[19]

Steroid supplementation may be required following adrenal disease or surgery for treatment of phaeochromocytoma. Local anaesthetics containing adrenaline (epinephrine) should be avoided. Consultation with a medical specialist is advisable.

## Musculoskeletal Disease

Patients with osteopetrosis (very rare) may be anaemic or taking corticosteroids which could affect surgical management. Radiotherapy to the head and neck often induces osteo-radionecrosis, which will delay healing and increases the risk of infection. Surgical treatment should only be carried out in a specialist centre. Aortic and mitral valve incompetence in Marfan's syndrome can lead to the risk of infective endocarditis, which may require antibiotic prophylaxis. The use of benzodi-azepine sedation is contraindicated in patients with myasthenia gravis due to the muscle-relaxant properties of this group of drugs.[20]

## Medication

### Non-Steroidal Anti-Inflammatory Drugs (NSAIDs)

Patients taking aspirin can suffer increased postoperative bleeding. However, aspirin therapy does not normally need to be stopped, and local haemostatic measures will normally control haemorrhage. Postoperative pain following surgery is often controlled with non-steroidal analgesics, which are contraindicated in patients taking warfarin due to enhancement of the anticoagulant effect. Non-steroidal drugs are nephrotoxic and should be avoided in renal disease. The toxicity of methotrexate, which is used for the treatment of rheumatoid arthritis, is greatly increased by combined therapy with NSAIDs.

### Warfarin

Patients taking warfarin should have their INR (international normalized ratio – a measure of the prothrombin time) measured within 24 hours of any surgical procedure. The normal therapeutic INR for patients on warfarin is 2.0–3.0, except for those with cardiac valve replacement, where the range is 2.5–4.0.[15] Current advice is that simple minor oral surgical procedures may be carried out if the INR is less than 3.0 without alteration of the warfarin dosage; block anaesthesia should be avoided if possible. If the INR is greater than 3.0, referral to the supervising physician or coagulation clinic is strongly advised.[18] There is evidence that patients are more likely to die from a thromboembolic problem as a result of reducing the drug than an uncontrolled bleed.[21] Drugs such as aspirin, diclofenac, diflunisal, ibuprofen and prolonged use of paracetamol all enhance the effect of warfarin. Erythromycin and metronidazole both increase the anticoagulant effects of warfarin and should be avoided.[18]

### Steroids

There is little evidence that steroid cover is required for general or surgical dental procedures under local anaesthetic.[15] For patients receiving long-term steroid medication in doses over 10 mg, it is sensible to double the usual dose on the day of treatment.[22]

## Liver and Kidney Disease

Patients with chronic renal disease will have reduced resistance to infection. Antibiotics should be prescribed following surgical dental procedures. These patients are often hypertensive and there may also be an increased risk of bleeding. Corticosteroids are often prescribed for these patients and an increased dose of medication may be required. Patients are best treated the day after dialysis, as platelet function will be optimal and the effect of the heparin will have worn off. Those with AV (arteriovenous) fistula should be given prophylactic antibiotics before dental procedures that cause a significant bacteraemia.[15] Consultation with the renal physician is advised.[23]

A patient with a history or signs that might suggest potential liver damage should have blood taken for liver function tests (LFTs) and clotting studies. Beware of the elderly patient with a penchant for sherry who has been prescribed NSAIDs for arthritis or aspirin for a heart complaint! Severe bleeding has been reported after dental extractions in patients with decompensated liver disease.[15] The liver is the main site for the metabolic removal of most local anaesthetics, and if metabolism is affected due to liver disease the plasma concentration will slowly increase. This may lead to signs of CNS toxicity with as little as 4 ml in an adult patient when liver disease is severe. The use of any drug in a patient with severe liver disease should be discussed with the patient's physician and checked in the BNF (British National

Formulary).[24] Erythromycin, metronidazole and tetracyclines should be avoided. NSAIDs increase the risk of gastrointestinal bleeding and interfere with fluid balance and are best avoided. Paracetamol is hepatotoxic and doses should be reduced.

### Gastrointestinal Disease

Patients with pancreatic disease, e.g. pancreatitis or pancreatic cancer, may have a bleeding tendency due to vitamin K malabsorption (pancreatitis) or biliary obstruction (cancer, especially if there are hepatic metastases). When the patient gives a history suggesting obstructive jaundice, the main risk in safe dental management relates to the risk of excessive bleeding, again resulting from vitamin K malabsorption.[25] When possible, surgery should be deferred. If delay is not possible, treatment in hospital with clotting factor supplementation is advised. NSAIDs should be avoided in patients with peptic ulcer disease, oesophagitis and gastritis, due to the increased risk of bleeding.[15]

### Pregnancy

During pregnancy, surgical endodontics is normally only considered in the mid-trimester and ideally should be avoided.

## Anatomical Factors

### Soft Tissues

#### Alveolar mucosa
The alveolar mucosa forms the sulcus and is loosely attached to the underlying tissue. The junction between alveolar mucosa and attached gingiva is known as the mucogingival junction. The quality of the mucosal tissue should be assessed prior to surgical treatment. When reflecting a flap where a long established sinus tract has been present, care must be taken to avoid tearing the friable mucosa (Figure 8.11).

#### Attached Gingiva
The attached gingiva is much more robust and is bound to the underlying bone. The blood

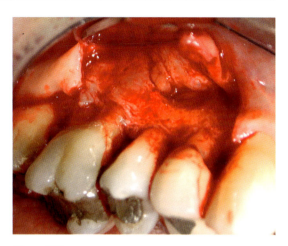

**Figure 8.11**

The maxillary second premolar was associated with chronic periapical periodontitis and a well-established sinus tract was present. On reflection of the flap, the tract can be seen firmly attached to the underside of the mucosa. It is important not to tear the friable mucosa, and sometimes the tissue will need to be separated from it using a pair of dissecting scissors or a scalpel blade.

supply to the alveolar mucosa and attached gingiva runs in a vertical direction. To reduce bleeding and avoid compromising the blood supply to a surgical flap, horizontal incisions are preferably avoided. The attached gingiva is assessed for colour, texture and vertical dimension. A wide band of attached gingiva may allow the use of a submarginal flap (Figure 8.12).

### Access and Size of the Oral Cavity

The ability of a patient to open the mouth and the size and shape of the oral cavity will influence the operator's view of the surgical site. A thick, prominent chin or mandibular buccal plate may present an increased density and depth of bone through which the operator will have to work. The height and depth of the vestibule is noted, as this will affect access. When there is little attached gingivae, the flap will encroach on the highly vascular alveolar mucosa. In this case it will be more difficult to elevate and retract. Also, access to the apical depth is restricted. This may lead to increased

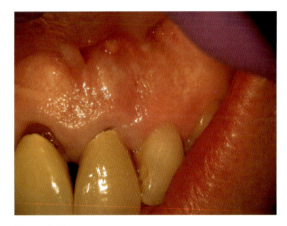

**Figure 8.12**

In this patient, there was a thick band of attached gingiva, which may lend itself to the use of a submarginal flap.

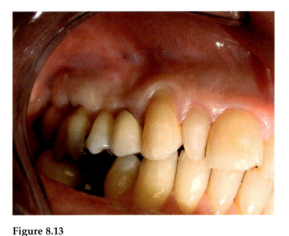

**Figure 8.13**

Root end surgery was considered in the posterior maxilla of this patient. Access is excellent, as the oral cavity is large and the sulcus deep. Good access will be provided to the roots of the maxillary premolars.

risk of bleeding during surgery, postoperative swelling and increased potential for ecchymosis. In contrast, a flap raised in a deep sulcus where there is a thick band of attached gingiva involves less connective tissue and is easier to incise, reflect and manage. This offers greater visibility and operating comfort once the flap is raised (Figure 8.13).

## Muscles and Frenal Attachments

The size, location and extent of any frenal attachments are noted. These may influence flap design.

## The Palate

The height and depth of the palate is examined. A deep palate allows much greater vertical access when using a palatal approach. A shallow palate not only presents visibility and elevation difficulties but also palatal root access is further complicated by the proximity of the greater palatine vessels. The palatal flap tends to be thick and challenging to retract during surgery. Reattachment of a palatal flap following surgery can also be problematic due to gravitational sagging and sometimes a stent may be required.

## Periodontal Status

Periodontal assessment prior to surgical endodontics is essential and periodontal probing should be carried out around the teeth in question. An assessment should be made of the likelihood of marginal adult periodontitis or the presence of a sinus tract in the gingival crevice. It may be necessary to carry out scaling and subgingival debridement prior to endodontic surgery and the patient should be given oral hygiene instruction. A narrow, deep pocket may indicate the presence of root fracture and therefore render the situation hopeless.

Loss of cortical bone from the buccal or lingual aspect that denudes the root surface has been shown to be a significant factor that has a negative effect on the outcome of endodontic surgery.[6] The success rate is further reduced when there is bone loss from both cortical plates.[26–28] Marginal periodontitis has been shown to be a significant factor in failure of root end surgery and persistence of periradicular inflammation.[10] It should be possible to detect the loss of cortical bone prior to surgery using careful periodontal probing. This will allow good presurgical assessment and planning. A dehiscence or fenestration that uncovers the root surface will dictate flap design and the level of root end resection. In some instances the use of bone regeneration techniques will be required (Figure 8.14).

## Restorability of the Tooth

Endodontic surgery would obviously not be considered if a tooth were not restorable or not considered important in the overall treatment plan.

## Buccal/Ridge

The extended width of the external oblique ridge in the mandible when combined with lingually placed apices will complicate visibility and access. Lip and cheek retraction is more difficult and uncomfortable in this region and, subsequently, postoperative surgical swelling and pain can be more extensive. Such problems may be solved by using an alternative treatment option such as extraction or referral to a more experienced colleague.

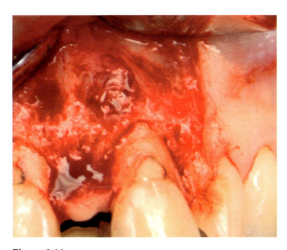

**Figure 8.14**

There has been significant pocketing around this maxillary incisor. A large lesion has perforated the cortical plate on the lateral border and there is virtually no remaining crestal bone on this part of the root surface. A submarginal flap would not be suitable in this instance as the horizontal incision will either run across the lesion or root surface and would not be situated on sound bone. A full-thickness flap is therefore required.

## Bony Exostoses

Large bony exostosis can make incision and raising of a flap considerably more difficult. The mucosa over them tends to be thin and can easily tear. Elevation, retraction and suturing are all more complicated.

## Neurovascular Anatomy

### The Inferior Dental Neurovascular Bundle (ID bundle)

Mandibular vessels travel anteriorly and buccally along the mandible to eventually end at the mental foramen. The bundle may be at risk during surgical treatment of mandibular molars and premolars. Usually, the neurovascular bundle lies inferior and lingual to the apices of the teeth.

Minor damage to the inferior dental nerve may result in anaesthesia. In some cases the nerve may reapproximate and reinnervate. Severing the artery within the bundle will cause immediate and extensive bleeding. The ID vessel can be located radiographically prior to treatment and if necessary a slice taken using an orthopantomogram (OPT) machine.

### Mental Bundle

Multiple periapical radiographs sometimes combined with an OPT will help the operator ascertain the location of the mental foramen. Its location will dictate where vertical incisions are made during flap reflection. Once the bundle is exposed, it should be kept visible throughout the surgery and protected from damage during reflection, bone removal or root resection. Bundle manipulation can leave the patient with minor tingling but it is extremely rare for the sensation to be long-lasting. Complete separation causes considerable bleeding and permanent lip anaesthesia. Should the nerve become completely severed, immediate referral to an oral surgeon may be necessary to ascertain whether reattachment is feasible. Reattachment can be very difficult as the nerve is usually under tension when the flap is reflected and snaps back into the foramen when severed. Uniting the two halves is therefore not always possible (Figure 8.15).

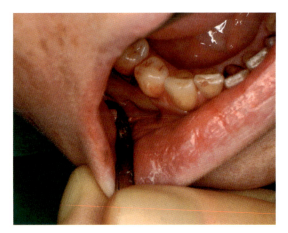

**Figure 8.15**

When carrying out surgery in the mandibular premolar region, it is essential to be aware of the position of the mental nerve. In this case it can be seen exiting from the mental foramen between the root apices of the mandibular premolars. Once the position has been established during root end surgery, a retractor should be placed above the superior margin so that damage cannot occur to it.

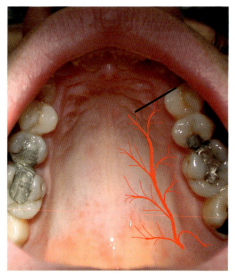

**Figure 8.16**

The palatine neurovascular bundle runs from the greater palatine foramen anteriorly (red). A relieving incision can be made mesial to the maxillary first premolar to avoid severing the bundle (black line).

*The Palatine Neurovascular Bundle*
The neurovascular bundle runs anteriorly from the greater palatine foramen approximately midway between the apex of the palatal vault and the gingival margin. It often lies in a bony canal. The bundle is vulnerable when using a palatal approach to the root apices. Vertical relieving incisions should not be made in the molar region, the flap should be raised carefully and the bundle protected during bone removal and root resection. A relieving incision can be made in the premolar/canine region (Figure 8.16).

*The Maxillary Sinus*
The maxillary sinus lies in close proximity to the root apices of the maxillary premolars and molars. The distance between the root tips and antrum varies and in some cases they may lie within the sinus, only separated by a thin membrane.

The proximity of the sinus does not preclude a particular tooth from surgery but it is generally considered advisable, if possible, to try to avoid perforating the antrum during apical surgery. Consequently, careful dissection is required during the procedure. The distance between the root apices and sinus can be estimated from a preoperative radiograph. If it is likely that the root apex is close or within the sinus, a more radical root resection may be required to prevent perforation of the antrum.

Occasionally, perforation cannot be avoided. In this case it is important to avoid displacing infected debris or the resected root tip into the maxillary sinus, as this can lead to the development of sinusitis.[29] The perforation is normally closed when the flap is replaced and there should be no risk of oroantral fistula formation and healing should be uneventful. Unlike the formation of a frank connection when a maxillary tooth is extracted, the prescription of an antral regimen consisting of antibiotics and antihistamines should not be required (Figure 8.17).

Individual Surgical Situations

*Maxillary Arch: Maxillary Incisors and Canine*
The root length of the central incisor is generally about 1–1.5 times the crown length and the

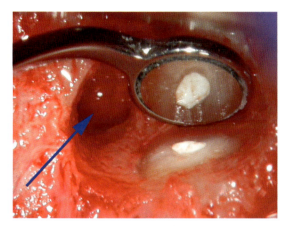

**Figure 8.17**

Due to the close proximity of the maxillary premolar root apices to the antrum, perforation will occasionally occur. In this case the maxillary antrum can be seen at the back of the osseous crypt (blue arrow). The defect will be closed when the flap is replaced and it is not normally necessary to prescribe an antral regimen.

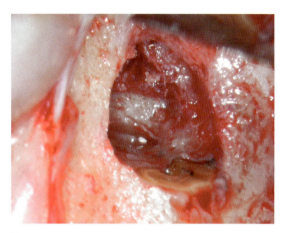

**Figure 8.18**

Access to the palatal root of maxillary premolars can be achieved from a buccal approach. However, when the roots are divergent the palatal root canal may be positioned a long way from the cortical plate. There is also an increased risk of perforating the antrum.

root apex is normally situated labially directly behind the cortical plate. Access is therefore relatively simple in most cases. The relationship between the root tip and the nasal floor is dependent on root length and the depth of the alveolar process. In some cases, a more coronal approach to the root apex will be required to prevent perforation of the nasal floor. Normally, a buccal approach is used. The root tip of the maxillary lateral incisor tends to be slender, deflecting both distally and in a palatal direction. When positioned distally, surgical access can be difficult. Occasionally, large lesions can be associated with the nasal floor and adequate local anaesthesia can be difficult to achieve. Developmental grooves on the palatal surface are sometimes present and can be associated with loss of cortical plate. Normally, a buccal approach is used.

*Maxillary Premolars and Molars*
The buccal root apices may be visible through a perforation in the cortical plate resulting from periapical pathology. The plate is generally thin and even when intact can often be perforated with a sharp probe in order to locate the root apex. Bone can be carefully removed using a sharp excavator to expose the root. In the first and second molar region the cortical plate can be thicker.

The palatal roots of the premolar and molar teeth may be approached from a buccal aspect using a transantral approach.[30] Although there have been few reports of difficulties using this technique, it is not particularly conservative and requires considerably more surgical expertise. The palatal roots of maxillary molars may be better identified using a palatal approach (Figure 8.18).

The roots of maxillary premolars are associated with an isthmus in approximately 30% of cases at the 3 mm level. The mesiobuccal root of the maxillary first molar commonly contains an isthmus.[31]

*Mandibular Incisors*
Access to the apices of the mandibular incisors can be one of the most challenging in surgical endodontics. Tooth angulation can result in the apex being positioned lingually and the cortical plate is often thick. The root tips are thin and close together. It can sometimes be difficult to avoid a bevel when resecting the root and there is often an isthmus at the apex. Injection of local anaesthetic into the mentalis muscle will result in increased bleeding (Figure 8.19).

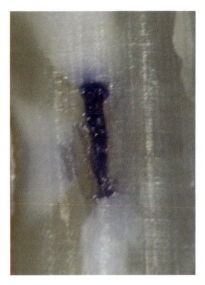

**Figure 8.19**

The resected root end of a mandibular incisor showing an isthmus. Due to the angulation of the mandibular incisors, it is not uncommon to have to bevel the root end slightly. This elongates the length of the isthmus that has to be prepared.

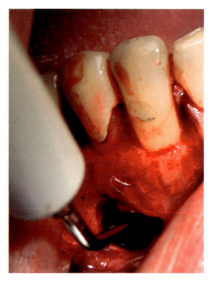

**Figure 8.20**

During root end surgery in the mandibular premolar region the mental nerve should be identified. Occasionally, the root end will need to be resected rather more aggressively to prevent damage to the nerve tissue.

*Mandibular Canine and Premolars*

The mental foramen should be identified; normally, the surgical approach is from a superior direction once the bundle has been identified. There are sometimes frenal and muscle attachments that may make reflection of the flap more difficult. Multiple canals are found in mandibular first premolars in approximately 33% of cases. These should be identified on a radiograph prior to surgery, as this will make surgical treatment more complex (Figure 8.20).

*Mandibular Molars*

Access to the mandibular root apices is more complex when the sulcus is shallow, the patient has a small oral cavity, the cortical plate is thick or the root apices are inclined lingually. The inferior dental canal must be identified on a radiograph. Sometimes a radiographic slice may be required. The canals in the mesial roots are very commonly connected by an isthmus,[32] which can often only be visualized using an operating microscope.[33] The more coronal resection of the mesial is carried out, the greater the chance of encountering an isthmus.[34] The isthmus will need to be cleaned and shaped during root end surgery. The roots can be wide in a buccolingual direction and inadequate root resection will fail to resect both canals. The use of an operating microscope is essential and methylene blue indicator dye may also help to identify the canals. It is essential that the operator is confident of the orientation and positioning of the apices prior to making osseous entry, as this avoids potential damage to adjacent teeth and prevents the osteotomy becoming excessively large. Using an operating microscope and microsurgical techniques has meant that surgery can now be completed very conservatively, with little tissue destruction (Figure 8.21).

*Clinical Assessment*

Clinical assessment includes a full medical and dental history, extraoral and intraoral examination, special investigations such as sensitivity testing, periodontal assessment and radiographs.

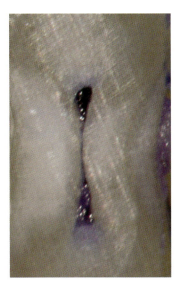

**Figure 8.21**

The isthmus between the mesial root canals in a mandibular molar will need to be cleaned using ultrasonics. An isthmus can be clearly seen in this case highlighted with canal blue indicator dye.

One of the aims of a clinical assessment is to minimize any procedural or healing complications that could occur by evaluating and recording the potential risks and difficulties prior to treatment.

Extraoral examination

- facial tissues and regional lymph nodes.

Intraoral examination

- general oral health
- presence of local infection
- swelling and sinus tracts
- the quality of restorations
- location of caries or cracks
- periodontal status, marginal periodontitis and pocketing
- sensitivity testing of the suspected tooth, adjacent teeth and its contralateral partner.

Radiological assessment

A long cone paralleling technique provides the best view of the tooth and the highest diagnostic yield. Usually, two views are taken to allow better assessment of the arrangement and orientation of the roots, any defects such as perforations and the size and positioning of periapical areas. If there is no lesion present, gaining access to the apex is not always obvious. It will need to be assessed from a measurement taken from the radiograph. At least 3 mm of the tissues at the apex of the roots should be included.[35] If a large periradicular lesion is suspected, a panoramic radiograph should be taken.

A gutta percha cone can be inserted into a sinus tract to delineate the tract on a radiograph. A sinus can sometimes track a considerable distance from the source. The presence of important anatomical landmarks such as the floor of the nose, the maxillary sinus, the mental foramen and inferior dental canal should also be noted. Historical radiographs can also be of value when assessing a case for surgery.

## REFERENCES

1. Danin J, Linder LE, Lundqvist G, Ohlsson L, Ramskold LO, Stromberg T. Outcomes of periradicular surgery in cases with apical pathosis and untreated canals. *Oral Surgery, Oral Medicine, Oral Pathology, Oral Radiology and Endodontics* 1999; **87:** 227–232.
2. Molven O, Halse A, Grung B. Observer strategy and the radiographic classification of healing after endodontic surgery. *International Journal of Oral and Maxillofacial Surgery* 1987; **16:** 432–439.
3. Andreasen JO, Rud J. Correlation between histology and radiography in the assessment of healing after endodontic surgery. *International Journal of Oral Surgery* 1972; **1:** 161–173.
4. Rud J, Andreasen JO, Möller Jensen JE. A follow-up study of 1000 cases treated by endodontic surgery. *International Journal of Oral Surgery* 1972; **1:** 215–228.
5. Molven O, Halse A, Grung B. Surgical management of endodontic failures: indications and treatment results. *International Dental Journal* 1991; **41:** 33–42.
6. Hirsh JM, Ahlström U, Henrikson PA, Heyden G, Peterson LE. Periapical surgery.

*International Journal of Oral Surgery* 1979; **8:** 173–185.

7. Mikkonen M, Kullaa-Mikkonen A, Kotilainen R. Clinical and radiologic re-examination of apicocectomized teeth. *Oral Surgery, Oral Medicine, Oral Pathology* 1983; **55:** 302–306.

8. Chong BS, Pitt Ford TR, Kariyawasam SP. Tissue response to potential root-end filling materials in infected canals. *International Endodontic Journal* 1997; **30:** 102–114.

9. Harrison JW, Jurosky KA. Wound healing in the tissues of the periodontium following periradicular surgery II. The dissectional wound. *Journal of Endodontics* 1991; **17:** 544–552.

10. Rud J, Andreasen JO. A study of failures after endodontic surgery by radiographic, histologic and stereomicroscopic methods. *International Journal of Oral Surgery* 1972; **1:** 311–328.

11. el-Swiah JM, Walker RT. Reasons for apicectomies. A retrospective study. *Endodontics and Dental Traumatology* 1996; **12:** 185–191.

12. Surgical Endodontic Guidelines: www.rcseng.ac.uk/dental/fds/pdf/surg_end_guideline.pdf

13. Nair PNR, Sjögren U, Krey G, Sunqvist G. Therapy-resistant foreign-body giant cell granuloma at the periapex of a root-filled human tooth. *Journal of Endodontics* 1990; **16:** 589–595.

14. Pitt Ford TR. Surgical treatment of apical periodontitis. In: Ørstavik D, Pitt Ford TR (eds). *Essential endodontics.* Oxford: Blackwell Science; 1998.

15. Sproat CP, Burke G, McGurk M. *Essentials of human disease for dentists.* Edinburgh: Elsevier; 2005.

16. Greenwood M, Meechan JG. General medicine and surgery for dental practitioners. Part 1: cardiovascular system. *British Dental Journal* 2003; **195:** 537–542.

17. Greenwood M, Meechan JG. General medicine and surgery for dental practitioners. Part 2: respiratory system. *British Dental Journal* 2003; **195:** 593–598.

18. Meechan JG, Greenwood M. General medicine and surgery for dental practitioners. Part 9: haematology and patients with bleeding problems. *British Dental Journal* 2003; **195:** 305–310.

19. Greenwood M, Meechan JG. General medicine and surgery for dental practitioners. Part 6: the endocrine system. *British Dental Journal* 2003; **195:** 129–133.

20. Greenwood M, Meechan JG. General medicine and surgery for dental practitioners. Part 8: musculoskeletal system. *British Dental Journal* 2003; **195:** 243–248.

21. Lockhart PB, Gibson J, Pond SH, Leitch J. Dental management considerations for the patient with an acquired coagulopathy. Part 1: coagulopathies from systemic disease. *British Dental Journal* 2003; **195:** 439–445.

22. Gibson N, Ferguson JW. Steroid cover for dental patients on long-term steroid medication: proposed clinical guidelines based upon a critical review of the literature. *British Dental Journal* 2004; **197:** 681–685.

23. Greenwood M, Meechan JG, Bryant DG. General medicine and surgery for dental practitioners. Part 7: renal disorders. *British Dental Journal* 2003; **195:** 181–184.

24. Greenwood M, Meechan JG. General medicine and surgery for dental practitioners. Part 5: liver disease. *British Dental Journal* 2003; **195:** 71–73

25. Greenwood M, Meechan JG. General medicine and surgery for dental practitioners. Part 3: gastrointestinal system. *British Dental Journal* 2003; **194:** 659–663.

26. Hirsh JM, Ahltrröm U, Henrikson PA, Heyden G, Petersen LE. Periapical surgery. *International Journal of Oral Surgery* 1979; **8:** 173–185.

27. Skoglund RF, Persson G. A follow-up study of apicoectomized teeth with total loss of the buccal bone plate. *Oral Surgery, Oral Medicine, Oral Pathology* 1985; **59:** 78–81.

28. Persson G. Periapical surgery of molars. *International Journal of Oral Surgery* 1982; **11:** 96–100.

29. Lin LL, Chance K, Shovlin F, Skribner J, Langeland K. Oroantral communication in periapical surgery of maxillary posterior teeth. *Journal of Endodontics* 1985; **11:** 40–44.

30. Wallace SM. Transantral endodontic surgery. *Oral Surgery, Oral Medicine, Oral*

*Pathology, Oral Radiology and Endodontics* 1996; **82:** 80–84.

31. Weller RN, Niemczyk SP, Kim S. Incidence and position of the canal isthmus. Part I. Mesiobuccal root of the maxillary first molar. *Journal of Endodontics* 1995; **21:** 380–383.

32. von Arx T. Frequency and type of canal isthmuses in first molars detected by endoscopic inspection during periradicular surgery. *International Endodontic Journal* 2005; **38:** 160–168.

33. Hsu YY, Kim S. The resected root surface. The issue of canal isthmuses. *Dental Clinics of North America* 1997; **41:** 529–540.

34. Cambruzzi JV, Marshall FJ. Molar endodontic surgery. *Journal of the Canadian Dental Association* 1983; **49:** 61–65.

35. Concensus report of the European Society of Endodontology on quality guidelines for endodontic treatment. *International Endodontic Journal* 1994; **27:** 115–124.

# 9 PAIN CONTROL, HAEMOSTASIS AND FLAP DESIGN

CONTENTS • Introduction • Placement of Anaesthetic • Surgical Equipment • Flap Design and Suturing • References

## INTRODUCTION

In order to carry out root end surgery, profound anaesthesia and tissue haemostasis are essential. Anaesthesia will eliminate any discomfort to the patient both during and immediately following surgery. Haemostasis improves vision at the surgical site and is essential in order to carry out effective root-end cavity preparation and filling. It will also help reduce post-surgical haemorrhage and swelling.

The local anaesthetic solution should contain a vasoconstrictor to achieve these objectives.[1] The vasoconstrictor serves two purposes: first, to retain the anaesthetic agent longer in the tissue, thereby extending the duration of anaesthetic; secondly, to enhance haemostasis. The most commonly used vasoconstrictor is adrenaline (epinephrine). Adrenaline causes vasoconstriction by stimulating membrane-bound $\alpha_1$ adrenergic receptors on the smooth muscle cells of blood vessels. These vessels are found in the oral tissues and skin. Adrenergic $\beta_1$ receptors in cardiac muscle induce increased heart rate, contractility and peripheral resistance. Blood vessels in skeletal muscles contain $\beta_2$ receptors which, when bound by adrenaline, cause vasodilation. This means that injection of adrenaline into muscle tissue will lead to increased blood flow and will have the opposite effect to that which is desired.[2]

Commercially available concentrations of vasoconstrictors in local anaesthetic solutions vary from 1:50 000 to 1:200 000. Although a concentration of 1:100 000 to 1:200 000 may be quite adequate for non-surgical treatment, it will not produce sufficient haemostasis for surgical procedures. For endodontic surgery, adrenaline at a concentration of at least 1:80 000 or 1:50 000 will be required for good haemostasis and visualization of the surgical site. Meeting these criteria will also reduce surgery time and decrease the risk of postoperative bleeding.[3]

The plasma concentrations of catecholamines and the haemodynamic responses to local anaesthetic solution containing 1:50 000 adrenaline were studied in dogs and it was concluded that the careful use of higher levels of a vasoconstrictor could be justified when patient profiles and surgical needs dictated.[4] The use of 2% lidocaine with adrenaline can elevate systemic plasma levels of adrenaline when used in high doses,[5,6] causing increased heart rate, cardiac contractility and peripheral vascular resistance in patients who are sensitive. These systemic reactions can be reduced by careful clinical assessment, surgical pre-planning and technique. The solution should not be injected intravascularly and the use of an aspirating syringe is recommended.

## PLACEMENT OF ANAESTHETIC

Local anaesthetic is infiltrated into the loose connective tissue of the alveolar mucosa near to the root apices. Placement too deep and into supraperiosteal tissues may result in increased bleeding due to the predominance of beta receptors in skeletal muscle. The anaesthetic will also be dispersed more rapidly in this situation and the duration of anaesthesia will therefore be reduced.

Local anaesthetic in volumes of 0.5 ml is normally deposited into numerous infiltration sites around the tooth that is to be treated. This ensures good anaesthesia and haemostasis. Injection should be carried out slowly at a rate of 1 or 2 ml/min.[7] Rapid injection produces pooling of anaesthetic in the tissues, which results in delayed diffusion and poor haemostasis (Figure 9.1).

## Maxillary Surgery

In the maxilla, buccal infiltration of 2–4 ml 2% lidocaine with 1:80 000 or 1:50 000 adrenaline is placed supraperiosteally into the submucosa over the apex of the tooth that is being treated. Increments of 0.5 ml are added mesially and distally. Palatal infiltration is obviously essential but can be uncomfortable even with mechanical delivery systems utilizing fine needles.[8] In the posterior quadrant, anaesthetic is deposited near to the greater palatine foramen to block the greater palatine nerve. The patient should be prewarned of the discomfort. Topical anaesthetic can be used but may not be totally effective in reducing discomfort.[8] A small amount of anaesthetic is deposited first and after 5 minutes the remainder injected very slowly. In the anterior region, anaesthetic is deposited into the incisive foramen to block the nasopalatine vessels. Occasionally, an inferior orbital block injection will be required for treatment in the maxillary canine or premolars. The anaesthetic is allowed to dissipate for at least 15 minutes prior to surgery, by which time the tissues should be blanched (Figure 9.2).

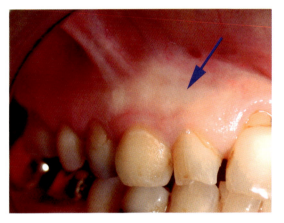

**Figure 9.1**

After approximately 15 minutes following infiltration of local anaesthetic, blanching of the tissues should be seen (blue arrow).

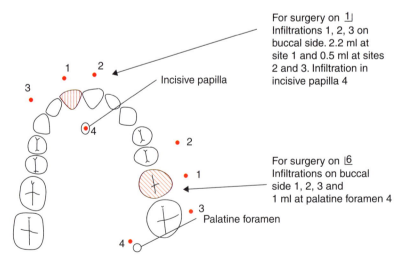

For surgery on 1⌋
Infiltrations 1, 2, 3 on buccal side. 2.2 ml at site 1 and 0.5 ml at sites 2 and 3. Infiltration in incisive papilla 4

Incisive papilla

For surgery on ⌊6
Infiltrations on buccal side 1, 2, 3 and 1 ml at palatine foramen 4

Palatine foramen

**Figure 9.2**

Anaesthesia for the maxillary arch.

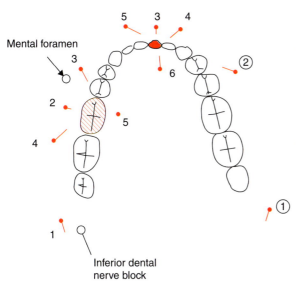

Anterior surgery: ⌐1
  1. Inferior dental nerve block and
     long buccal infiltration
  2. Mental nerve infiltration
  3. Infiltration buccal 3, 4, 5
  4. Infiltration lingual 6

Posterior surgery: ⌐6
  1. Inferior dental nerve block and
     long buccal infiltration
  2. Infiltration buccal 2, 3, 4
  3. Infiltration lingual 5

**Figure 9.3**

Anaesthesia for the mandibular arch.

## Mandibular Surgery

In the mandible, a mandibular nerve block and long buccal infiltration will be required, for which local anaesthetic containing 1:100 000 adrenaline can be used. Supplemental infiltrations will then be required with at least 1:80 000 adrenaline.[9] Local anaesthetic is deposited adjacent to the root apex of the tooth that is to be treated and then mesially, distally and lingually. Again, a period of at least 15 minutes is allowed for the anaesthetic to take effect, by which time the gingival tissues should be blanched. It is essential to achieve predictable anaesthesia prior to commencing surgery, as attempts to regain it during surgery can be difficult (Figure 9.3).

## Pre-emptive Analgesia

Preoperative, non-steroidal anti-inflammatory drugs (NSAIDs) may prevent postoperative pain.[10] Pre-emptive analgesia is administered on the basis that the drug will be present in a therapeutic dose prior to pain developing rather than being required in response to it.

This strategy has been shown to be effective in reducing pain during the postoperative period and results in fewer analgesics being required.[11] Both NSAIDs or the relatively newer cyclooxygenase-2 (COX-2) inhibiting drugs should be effective in suppressing pain immediately following surgery but may also prevent peripheral and central sensitization which can lead to hyperalgesia.[12] An effective approach in managing moderate to severe postoperative endodontic pain is to administer NSAIDs and a paracetamol–opioid in combination.[13]

## Long-acting Anaesthesia

Long-acting anaesthetics such as bupivacaine provide postoperative analgesia for up to 8–10 hours following block injection. They may help reduce postoperative pain (Figure 9.4).[14,15]

## SURGICAL EQUIPMENT

Most practitioners create a bespoke kit of surgical instruments with elements from different sources. The basic surgical requirements

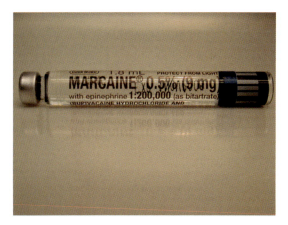

**Figure 9.4**

Marcaine (bupivacaine hydrochloride) is a long-acting local anaesthetic which can be used to help reduce postoperative pain.

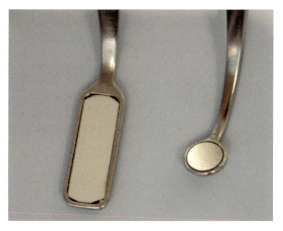

**Figure 9.6**

Surgical mirrors can be made of stainless steel or glass. Metal mirrors have to be handled with care to avoid scratching of the mirrored surface (J&S Davis).

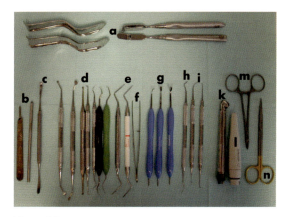

**Figure 9.5**

A basic surgical kit: (a) retractors; (b) standard surgical and microsurgical handle for scalpel blades; (c) periosteal elevator; (d) curettes; (e) root tip elevators; (f) rat-tooth tweezers; (g) sapphire glass retro mirrors; (h) fine flat plastic; (i) burnishers and pluggers; (k) high-speed surgical handpiece; (l) Piezon ultrasonic handpiece; (m) suture holders; and (n) suture scissors.

are divided into the following categories (Figures 9.5–9.10):

- Incision:
  Standard and microscalpel holders and blades
- Reflection of flap:
  Periosteal elevator
  Flap retractors

- Penetration of bone:
  High-speed surgical handpiece with reverse exhaust
  Low-speed straight surgical handpiece with water coolant
  Bone burs
  Probe
  Curettes
- Excision or curetting of lesion:
  A series of graded curettes and periodontal instruments
  Locking and rat-tooth tweezers
- Root end resection:
  Long diamond and tungsten carbide straight fissure burs
- Root end preparation:
  Micromirrors
  Ultrasonic Piezon unit
  Ultrasonic root end tips
- Root end filling:
  Carrier
  Pluggers
  Burnisher
- Irrigation:
  Large syringe, wide-bore needle and sterile saline
- Flap replacement:
  Assorted sutures
  Needle holders
  Scissors

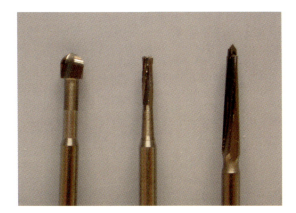

**Figure 9.7**

A round surgical bur, a fissure bur and Lindemann bur can all be used with a high-speed surgical handpiece for bone removal and root end resection.

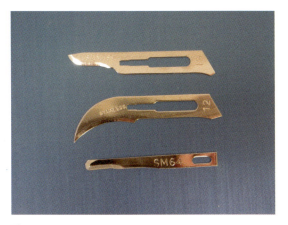

**Figure 9.8**

Surgical blades Nos 12 and 15 are useful for most incisions. Blade No. 15 is used for vertical relieving incisions while No. 12 is useful for interproximal areas. Microsurgical blades are also available.

- Miscellaneous:
  Surgical suction tip
  Microsuction tips
  Stropko irrigator
  Methylene blue
  Haemostatic materials
  Swabs
  Root-end filling material MTA, Super EBA, IRM
  Histopathology pot and formal saline.

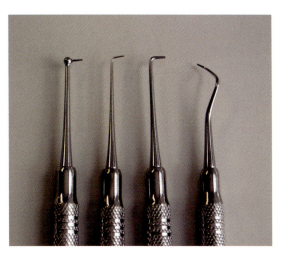

**Figure 9.9**

There are various pluggers available for packing root-end filling material. Different sizes will be required and a curette (right-hand side) is useful for removing excess material.

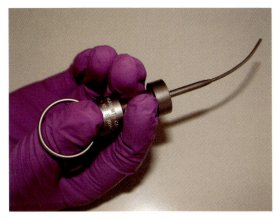

**Figure 9.10**

The Dovgan MTA gun can be used to deposit filling material into the root end cavity. Unfortunately, this design can become easily blocked and needs to be cleaned with care.

## FLAP DESIGN AND SUTURING

### Introduction

Access for root end surgery should provide sufficient visibility of the surgical field and any associated pathology. Flap design is critical to ensure good surgical access and postoperative healing.

## Preoperative Disinfection

A preoperative mouth rinse of 0.2% chlorhexidine gluconate has been recommended,[16,17] as this improves postoperative healing by preventing the risk of infection. This can be started 24 hours prior to surgery but can also be swilled for 1 minute prior to placement of anaesthetic. Patients should be advised to refrain from smoking, and if sedation is used they must bring an accompanying person who will be responsible for escorting them home and ensuring compliance with all postoperative instructions.

## Flap Design

Full mucoperiosteal flaps should be used for endodontic surgery whenever possible as they perform well from a biological perspective, offer excellent surgical access and ensure good tissue healing. The flap may have a horizontal boundary in the gingival crevice or submarginally.

## Full-Thickness Marginal Flaps with One or Two Relieving Incisions

### Horizontal Flap

The horizontal flap consists of an incision that runs along the gingival sulcus. The scalpel blade is held as near to vertical as possible and interdentally the papilla is severed at the mid-col position. A No. 12 blade is useful in this area. A No. 15 scalpel blade or microsurgical blade can be used around the tooth margins. The horizontal flap can be used for investigation of the root surface – e.g. when looking for root fractures – but gives restricted access to the root tip. In this case, a vertical relieving incision will be required and the flap then becomes triangular (one relieving incision) or rectangular (two relieving incisions).

### Full-Thickness Triangular and Rectangular Flaps

A primary incision is made in the gingival sulcus and follows the contours of the teeth.

Sufficient space must be provided either side of any intrabony pathology to prevent the relieving incision lying over the defect and potentially affecting healing. The relieving incision is started at the gingival margin and extends through the attached gingiva. The incision should be made with a firm continuous stroke and the blade not lifted from the bone until the incision is complete. This avoids jagged edges, which are difficult to suture. Extension deep into the sulcus is not required and can lead to increased bleeding into the operative site. Normally, the papilla is preserved. One relieving incision (triangular full-thickness flap) may give sufficient visibility. However, two relieving incisions (rectangular full-thickness flap) will provide much greater surgical access. From a biological perspective, relieving incisions should be as vertical as possible to avoid severing supraperiosteal vessels and collagen fibres. This will reduce bleeding and improve healing. They should be positioned in root concavities between bony eminences. The mucoperiosteal tissue is always thinner over eminences and is much more difficult to suture. Healing is normally by primary intention, and providing there is good oral hygiene postoperative problems are minimal.[18] One disadvantage is that the horizontal incision in the gingival crevice has been associated with postoperative gingival recession,[19,20] but this may not always be a significant factor.[21]

Some authors have recommended a modification known as the papilla base incision to preserve the papilla and reduce postoperative recession (Figures 9.11–9.20).[22,23]

### Submarginal Flap (Luebke–Ochsenbein)

This submarginal flap is best used in cases where there is a thick band of attached gingiva. The horizontal incision is contained within the attached gingiva and is scalloped to mimic the gingival margin. A minimum of 3 mm of gingival tissue should be retained coronally to prevent ischaemia, necrosis and sloughing of the band of gingiva. One or more relieving incisions are then made to reflect the flap.[24] The flap is not really suitable for use in

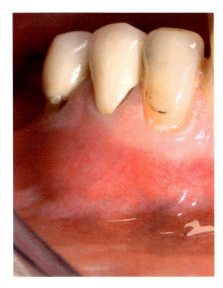

**Figure 9.11**

Root end surgery was required on this mandibular first premolar. A full-thickness triangular flap will be used with a relieving incision mesial to the mandibular canine.

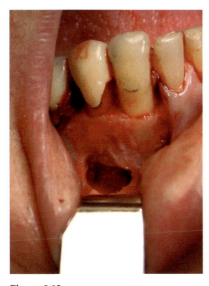

**Figure 9.12**

Good visibility and access has been achieved for the root end of the mandibular first premolar. The borders of the flap will be on sound bone when replaced.

the mandible. It can be very useful in the anterior maxilla, especially if the gingival tissue has to be preserved adjacent to crowned teeth (Figures 9.21–9.23).[25]

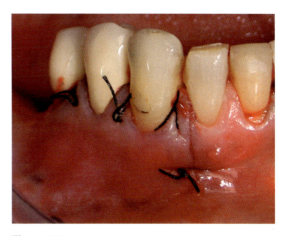

**Figure 9.13**

Immediately following flap replacement. Four black silk sutures have been used to retain the flap.

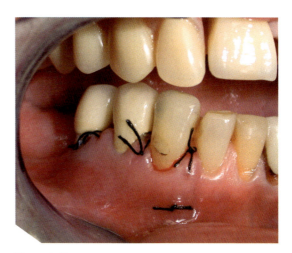

**Figure 9.14**

Three days later, the sutures were removed. Using chlorhexidine gluconate mouthwash reduces inflammation and good primary healing has occurred.

## Palatal Flaps

A full-thickness flap with one or two relieving incisions gives the best access. The anterior relieving incision is made at the mesiolingual line angle of the first premolar and extends two-thirds of the distance to the apex of the palatal vault. If a distal relieving incision is required, this should be made from the distal line angle of the last molar and is extended posteriorly along the pad. There is high risk of

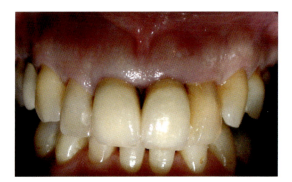

**Figure 9.15**

There is a large periapical lesion around the apices of the upper left central and lateral incisor. A rectangular flap will be required to gain surgical access.

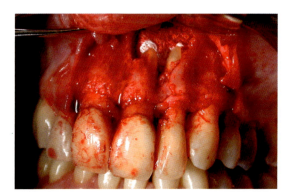

**Figure 9.16**

The rectangular flap has been designed so that good visibility can be achieved. The lesion associated with these teeth is large and extends superiorly to the floor of the nose. The boundaries of the flap will lie on sound bone when it is replaced.

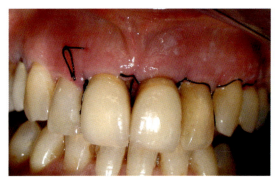

**Figure 9.17**

At the suture removal appointment 3 days later excellent primary healing can be seen. There is little evidence of inflammation around the sutures.

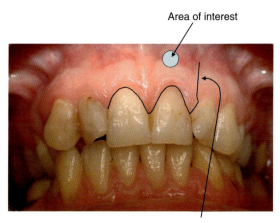

Area of interest

The relieving incision meets the gingival crevice at 90 degrees and runs vertically upwards

**Figure 9.18**

Triangular flap.

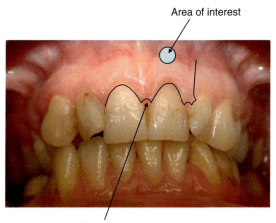

Area of interest

Papilla base incision to preserve the papilla

**Figure 9.19**

Triangular flap.

severing the palatine neurovascular bundle if a lingually inclined relieving incision is used in the posterior region.

The periosteal elevator must be guided across the bone of the palatal vault, but reflection of the flap can be difficult as the tissues are leathery and firmly bound. A sling suture can aid retraction of the flap (Figures 9.24–9.26).

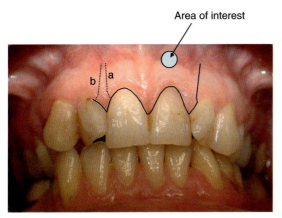

Relieving incision "a" papilla intact
Relieving incision "b" papilla retracted

**Figure 9.20**

Rectangular flap.

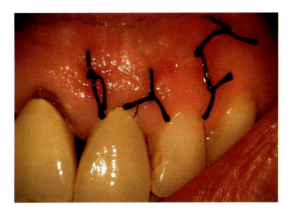

**Figure 9.22**

Three days later, there is good evidence of healing by primary intention.

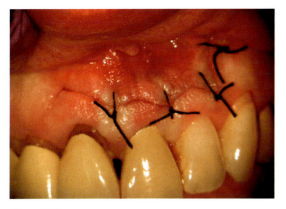

**Figure 9.21**

In this case a Luebke–Ochsenbein flap was raised. The flap has been sutured using silk sutures.

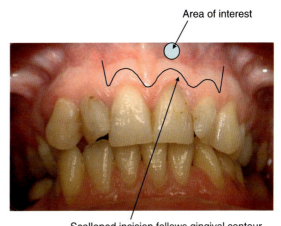

Scalloped incision follows gingival contour

**Figure 9.23**

Luebke–Ochsenbein flap.

## Semilunar Flap

Semilunar flaps tend to be associated with more postoperative problems and scarring and are therefore contraindicated for use in root end surgery (Figure 9.27).[18,19,26]

## Reflecting the Flap

The periosteal elevator should have a keen, undamaged blade to ensure atraumatic reflection of the flap. The instrument is first inserted into the relieving incision at the level of the attached gingiva. It is passed under the periosteum to reflect the tissues and moved gently in a lateral direction, maintaining contact with the cortical bone. The periosteum and superficial tissues are reflected from the cortical plate. The papillae are reflected by moving the elevator coronally, undermining the gingivae.[18] Tags of tissue will be seen on the surface of the cortical bone. These are retained as they will help reattachment of the flap and also aid healing (Figures 9.28, 9.29).

## Retraction

The flap should be retracted so that tissue damage is minimized. The retractor should

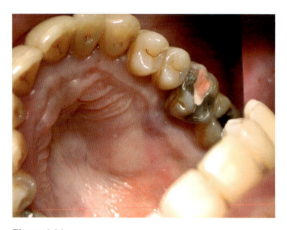

**Figure 9.24**

Palatal access is required to the maxillary first molar. A full-thickness flap will be raised with a relieving incision mesial to the maxillary first premolar.

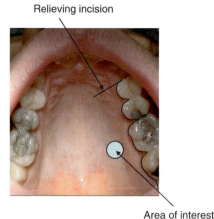

**Figure 9.26**

Palatal flap.

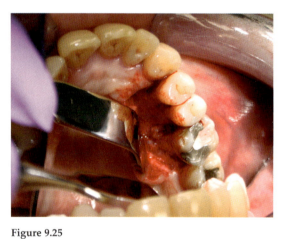

**Figure 9.25**

The flap has been raised. Due to the thickness of the palatal mucosa, the flap can be difficult to retract and access is sometimes limited.

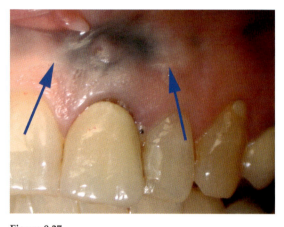

**Figure 9.27**

Scarring from previous surgery using a semilunar flap can be seen (blue arrows). Unfortunately, root end surgery using an amalgam retrograde technique has failed and this has resulted in an amalgam tattoo. There is a draining buccal sinus tract associated with the maxillary left central incisor.

rest on bone and not pinch the soft tissues. If insufficient access is created, the marginal or relieving incisions may need to be extended.

## Replacement of the Flap

The flap is gently eased into place and gentle pressure applied for 2–3 minutes prior to suturing. This brings the tissue tags on the bony surface and underside of the gingival flap into close approximation for reattachment. Suturing will nearly always be necessary, following which pressure is again applied for 5–10 minutes. This ensures good adaptation of the flap to the underlying bone and helps prevent haemorrhage occurring and mitigates against potential infection.[27] Postoperative care will be discussed in Chapter 10 (Figure 9.30).

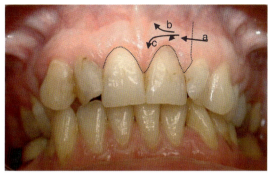

Reflection of the flap starts at the relieving incision and proceeds in the order:

a–b–c working laterally across the flap

**Figure 9.28**

Flap reflection.

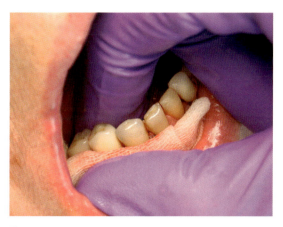

**Figure 9.30**

Pressure is applied to the flap following replacement to initiate good adaptation and help reduce haemorrhage.

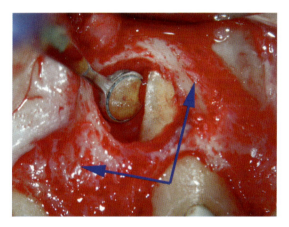

**Figure 9.29**

Tissue tags (blue arrows) are present on the cortical bone surface. They will help reattachment of the flap and also healing following surgery.

## Sutures

Sutures are required to hold the tissue flap in position and prevent dislodgement, thereby allowing healing by primary intention.

Many different materials have been suggested. Braided or multistrand sutures such as those made of silk can become infected with bacterial plaque that wicks along the material when exposed to the oral environment. It is necessary to use an antibacterial mouthwash such as chlorhexidine gluconate while the

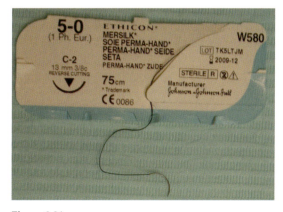

**Figure 9.31**

A gauge 5/0 silk suture.

sutures are in place to prevent them becoming infected, which results in localized inflammation.[17] The sutures are normally removed after 48–72 hours,[18] at which point early epithelialization will have occurred. If silk sutures are left in situ for too long, there is a risk of damage to the dental papilla (Figure 9.31).[25]

Single-strand or monofilament sutures such as polyglactin, polypropylene, polyethylene or Teflon (polytetrafluoroethylene) result in no bacterial wicking and little inflammation but can sometimes be more difficult to place (Figures 9.32, 9.33).

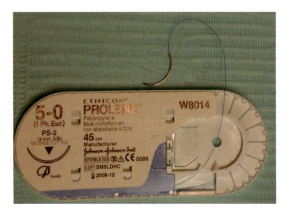

**Figure 9.32**

Monofilament sutures such as polypropylene can be very useful in endodontic surgery. There is no risk of bacterial wicking and the suture is relatively easy to use. The cut ends can be prickly on the buccal mucosa.

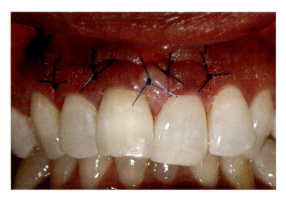

**Figure 9.33**

A Prolene (polypropylene) monofilament suture has been used to retain a Luebke–Ochsenbein flap with interrupted sutures. The sutures will be removed in 3 days. A minor frenectomy has also been carried out in this case.

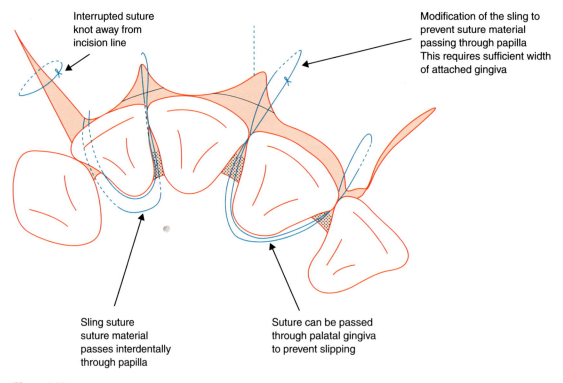

**Figure 9.34**

Interrupted and sling sutures.

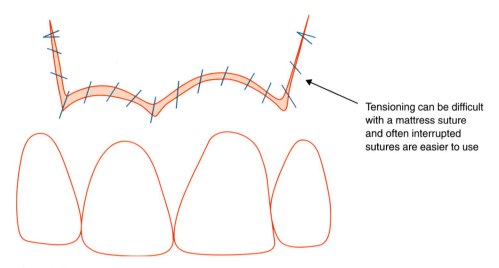

**Figure 9.35**

Mattress suture.

A variety of sutures sizes 4/0 to 6/0, with various curvatures and radii of needle are used, depending on the anatomical situation.

The minimum number of sutures that are required to retain the flap should be used. Interrupted sutures are frequently used to retain a full-thickness flap. They can be modified to provide a sling, thereby avoiding having to place the suture material through the papilla (Figure 9.34).

Mattress sutures have been advocated for securing partial-thickness flaps. However, there can be difficulties with tensioning, when using this technique (Figure 9.35).

Tensioning can be difficult with a mattress suture and often interrupted sutures are easier to use

## REFERENCES

1. Jastak JT, Yagiela JA. Vasoconstrictors and local anaesthesia: a review and rationale for use. *Journal of the American Dental Association* 1983; **107**: 623–630.
2. Milam SB, Giovannitti JA Jr. Local anaesthetics in dental practice. *Dental Clinics of North America* 1984; **28**: 493–508.
3. Buckley JA, Ciancio SG, McMullen JA. Efficacy of epinephrine concentration in local anesthesia during surgery. *Journal of Periodontology* 1984; **55**: 653–657.
4. Gutmann JL, Frazier LW, Baron B. Plasma catecholamine and haemodynamic responses to surgical endodontic anaesthetic protocols. *International Endodontic Journal* 1996; **29**: 37–42.
5. Troullos ES, Goldstein DS, Hargreaves KM, Dionne RA. Plasma epinephrine levels and cardiovascular response to high administered doses of epinephrine contained in local anaesthesia. *Anaesthesia Progress* 1987; **34**: 10–13.
6. Hasse AL, Heng MK, Garrett NA. Blood pressure and electrocardiographic response to dental treatment and the use of local anaesthesia. *Journal of the American Dental Association* 1986; **113**: 639–642.
7. Roberts DH, Sowray JH. *Local analgesia in dentistry*, 2nd edn. Bristol: Wright; 1987.
8. Nusstein J, Burns Y, Reader A, Beck M, Weaver J. Injection pain and postinjection pain of the palatal-anterior superior alveolar injection, administered with the Wand Plus system, comparing 2% lidocaine with 1:100,000 epinephrine to 3% mepivacaine. *Oral Surgery, Oral Medicine, Oral Pathology, Oral Radiology and Endodontics* 2004; **97**: 164–172.
9. Kim S, Edwall L, Trowbridge H, Chien S. Effects of local anaesthetics on pulpal blood flow in dogs. *Journal of Dental Research* 1984; **63**: 650–652.

10. Jackson DL, Moore PA, Hargreaves KM. Preoperative nonsteroidal anti-inflammatory medication for the prevention of postoperative dental pain. *Journal of the American Dental Association* 1989; **119**: 641–646.

11. Dionne RA. Preemptive vs preventative analgesia: which approach improves clinical outcomes? *Compendium of Continuing Education in Dentistry* 2000; **21**: 51–54.

12. Khan AA, Dionne RA. COX-2 inhibitors for endodontic pain. *Endodontic Topics* 2002; **3**: 31–40.

13. Hargreaves KM, Baumgartner JC. *Principles and practice of endodontics*, 3rd edn. Philadelphia: WB Saunders; 2002.

14. Keiser K, Hargreaves KM. Building effective strategies for the management of endodontic pain. *Endodontic Topics* 2002; **3**: 93–105.

15. Moore PA. Bupivacaine: a long-lasting local anesthetic for dentistry. *Oral Surgery, Oral Medicine, Oral Pathology* 1984; **58**: 369–374.

16. Martin MV, Nind D. Use of chlorhexidine gluconate for pre-operative disinfection of apicectomy sites. *British Dental Journal* 1987; **162**: 459–461.

17. Tsesis I, Fuss Z, Lin S, Tilinger G, Peled M. Analysis of postoperative symptoms following surgical endodontic treatment. *Quintessence International* 2003; **34**: 756–760.

18. Gutmann JL, Harrison JW. *Surgical endodontics*. St Louis: Ishiyaku EuroAmerica; 1994.

19. Kramper BJ, Kaminski EJ, Osetek EM, Heuer MA. A comparative study of the wound healing of three types of flap design used in periapical surgery. *Journal of Endodontics* 1984; **10**: 17–25.

20. Velvart P, Ebner-Zimmermann U, Pierre Ebner J. Papilla healing following sulcular full thickness flap in endodontic surgery. *Oral Surgery, Oral Medicine, Oral Pathology, Oral Radiology and Endodontis* 2004; **98**: 365–369.

21. Harrison JW, Jurosky KA. Wound healing in the tissues of the periodontium following periradicular surgery II. The dissectional wound. *Journal of Endodontics* 1991; **17**: 544–552.

22. Velvart P. Papilla base incision: a new approach to recession-free healing of the interdental papilla after endodontic surgery. *International Endodontic Journal* 2002; **35**: 453–460.

23. Velvart P, Ebner-Zimmermann U, Ebner JP. Comparison of papilla healing following sulcular full-thickness flap and papilla base flap in endodontic surgery. *International Endodontic Journal* 2003; **36**: 653–659.

24. Luebke RG. Surgical endodontics. *Dental Clinics of North America* 1974; **18**: 379–391.

25. Grung B. Healing of gingival mucoperiosteal flaps after marginal incision in apicoectomy procedures. *International Journal of Oral Surgery* 1973; **2**: 20–25.

26. Gutmann JL. Principles of endodontic surgery for the general practitioner. *Dental Clinics of North America* 1984; **28**: 895–908.

27. Hiat WH, Stallard RE, Butler ED, Badget B. Repair following mucoperiosteal flap surgery with full gingival retention. *Journal of Periodontology* 1968; **39**: 11–16.

# 10 SURGICAL PROCEDURES

## INTRODUCTION

Endodontic surgical procedures include:

- curettage
- apicectomy
- root amputation
- hemisection
- perforation repair.

Following reflection of a suitable flap, the operative field can be visualized. Root end surgery is probably the most common surgical endodontic procedure.

## PENETRATION OF THE CORTICAL PLATE

Following reflection of the flap, the location of the root tip is estimated. If the tooth has been associated with a large periapical lesion, the cortical plate will often have been perforated (Figures 10.1, 10.2).

A sharp excavator can be used to reflect the thin bone around the perforation to improve visibility and access. The instrument is then introduced into the bony crypt in an attempt to currette the lesion intact.[1] If the cortical plate has not been perforated by expansion of underlying pathology, bone will need to be removed to expose and identify the root apex. Bone removal can be carried out using a surgical round bur in a straight handpiece with sterile irrigant or with a high-speed handpiece such as the Phatelus 45 (NSK, Kanuma, Tochigi, Japan). The head of the latter handpiece

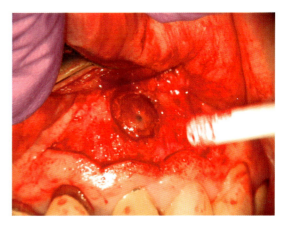

**Figure 10.1**

The cortical plate has been perforated by expansion of this radicular cyst.

is angled at 45° and the exhaust air ejected away from the surgical site. Tungsten carbide or steel burs are used in preference to diamond burs for bone removal as they are less likely to clog with bone fragments and generate heat. An estimate of the root length can be made from a paralleling radiograph and transferred directly onto the exposed bone using a periodontal probe. Bone is carefully removed using a light brush stroke action with the bur. When viewed under the microscope, it is much easier to identify the underlying root surface, but great care must be taken not to damage the cementum layer as this could result in resorption. The root is normally encountered in a more coronal position, and bone is carefully removed in an apical direction until the lesion

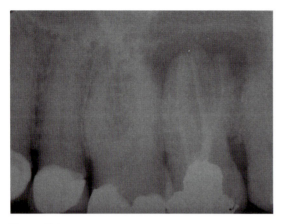

**Figure 10.2**

There is a very large radiolucency associated with the maxillary second molar. Non-surgical retreatment would be carried out first, as it is quite likely that the root canals are infected. The lesion undoubtedly perforates the maxillary sinus and is very large. Surgery in this instance may be better carried out under general anaesthetic in a hospital environment.

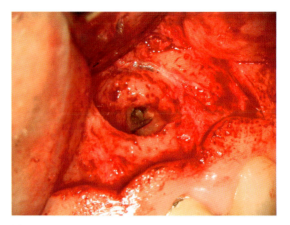

**Figure 10.3**

The radicular cyst has been curetted in one piece and the bony cavity remains.

is uncovered. The osseous window is then enlarged until sufficient space is provided to give adequate access for curettage. The root can be identified from bone by its texture and colour, the root surface being smooth and yellow, and the fact that it does not bleed.

## CURETTAGE

Curettage involves the removal of reactive soft tissue from around the root end with or without root end resection and cavity preparation. Curettage is normally carried out when there has been no evidence of healing following root canal treatment or retreatment. As most periapical lesions are the result of an inflammatory response to bacterial infection within the root canal, removal of a lesion without cleaning the root canal system will undoubtedly result in failure. Curettage may also be used either to remove extruded materials that are causing an inflammatory response or in a situation where a biopsy is required. There has been some debate as to whether it is necessary to remove all the remnants of a soft tissue lesion. Indeed some of the tissue remnants at the borders of a

lesion could be responsible for initiating the healing process. Most of the irritants will be contained within the root canal, and therefore complete curettage should not be necessary. Clinical evidence has shown no statistical difference at follow-up appointments between cases where complete curettage and incomplete removal of periapical tissues had been achieved.[2] In cases where a lesion lies in close proximity to vulnerable anatomical tissues, priority should be given to preserving the vital structures.[2] In situations involving *Actinomyces* infection, in which the microorganisms can survive in the extraradicular environment by clumping together, the lesion would have a granular yellow appearance and should ideally be completely and carefully excised during surgery if at all possible.

Curettage is normally carried out with a straight or angled surgical bone curette or a periodontal curette. The curette is first worked around the margins of the lesion, with the convex surface innermost to reflect the lesion from the surrounding bone. The curette is then reversed to scoop out the soft tissue lesion (Figures 10.3, 10.4).[1]

Removing this tissue helps to reduce bleeding should further treatment be required and will also help to reduce the chances of postoperative haemorrhage. Any lesion that is removed should be immediately placed in formal saline and sent for histopathological examination.[3] If the lesion cannot be removed

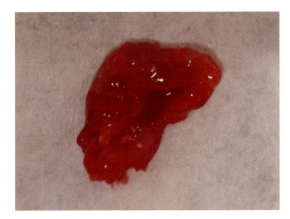

**Figure 10.4**

A lesion has been curetted and will be sent for histopathological analysis.

in one piece, fragments are retained and examined individually. If a lesion is very large and extends over the root apices of adjacent teeth, care must be taken to avoid compromising the neurovascular bundle, which could potentially result in these teeth becoming non-vital. Inadvertent penetration of a lesion during surgery may lead to increased bleeding or in *Actinomyces* lesions, the release of microorganisms into the surgical site. Tissue can be quite firmly attached to the root surface and a well-honed periodontal curette will be required to remove it without damaging the root surface. Sometimes, even with profound anaesthesia, the patient can be aware of discomfort when a lesion is being removed. This may be as a result of increased neural budding within the centre of a lesion that has been stimulated by inflammatory mediators.[4] Injecting local anaesthetic into the lesion over a few minutes will normally resolve the problem. Curettage is normally carried out prior to treatment of the root end.

## APICECTOMY

### Root End Resection

The root end is resected in order to identify the root canal and provide access to the source of infection. Historically, resection and bevelling was carried out in order to improve access to the root canal for preparation with a round bur.[5] The apex of most teeth contains multiple foramina and by removing the apical 2–3 mm of the root most of these can be removed,[6] but care must be taken not to compromise the crown-to-root length ratio.

Current biological evidence and advances in preparation techniques, such as the use of ultrasonic surgical tips with an operating microscope, have meant that the angle of bevel should be reduced. Bevelling exposes dentinal tubules, which can allow the leakage of bacterial byproducts and irritants from the root canal past the root end filling.[7,8] In older patients, there will have been greater intertubular sclerosis and this reduces the patency of dentinal tubules.[9,10] The root is therefore resected perpendicular to the root canal to reduce the number of exposed dentinal tubules.[11] The root surface is then checked for smoothness, cracks and canal irregularities (Figure 10.5).[12,13]

When resecting the root, smear will be produced on the cut root surface. This could potentially be infected and theoretically delay or prevent healing. Smear is more likely to be produced when a course diamond bur has been used or when cutting without water spray. A diamond bur of medium, fine or ultrafine grade, or a tungsten carbide bur is recommended for resection and should be used with coolant water spray. This will prevent tissue damage and reduce the production of smear and snagging of the root filling material (Figure 10.6).[14]

If access is good, the tip of the root can be reduced by planing from the apex and cutting coronally. A straight tungsten carbide fissure bur or a Lindemann bone bur can be used in a high-speed handpiece. This method allows a very precise removal of tooth substance and is continued until the root canal can be visualized. An alternative approach is to assess the amount of root tip to be removed, place the bur lateral to the root at this level and section it. This technique may be useful when the root is in close proximity to important anatomical features such as the sinus lining, inferior dental canal or mental nerve. However, this method invariably results in a greater portion of root being resected. Once the root apex has been removed, the cut surface can be polished

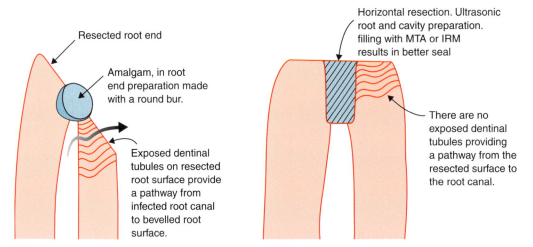

**Figure 10.5**

Root end resection.

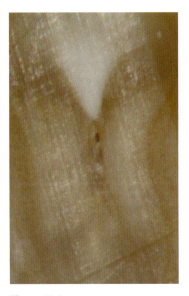

**Figure 10.6**

The resected root end has a rough appearance when a diamond bur is used.

with a fine tungsten carbide or a diamond bur but there is no evidence to show that any particular bur provides a better outcome following resection. The level to which the root end is resected will be dictated by many factors such as the degree of visibility achieved at the surgical site, the positioning of the root tip within the crypt and the position of vulnerable anatomical structures. Originally, the root was resected at the base of a large periapical lesion. In theory this was to remove potentially infected root substance but is no longer considered appropriate or necessary.[15] In multiple rooted teeth, it may be necessary to reduce the buccal roots slightly to give adequate access to a lingually based canal. If the bony crypt is small, or the soft tissues restrict reflection of the flap reducing access, then further reduction of the root may be required in order to make enough space for root end preparation. Alternatively, the crypt may be enlarged. In situations where perforation repair is required, the level of resection may be dictated by the positioning and level of a perforation. In cases where there has been marginal bone loss as a result of periodontal disease, leaving less than 1 mm of crestal bone on the buccal aspect of the root could seriously affect the outcome of treatment. Once the root has been resected, an inspection is carried out with the operating microscope at high magnification or using a microendoscope. Sometimes, small knife edges of root may be retained on the lateral borders, or if the root is angled, it may not have been adequately severed to expose the root canals (Figures 10.7–10.9).

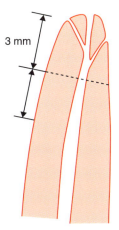

The apical 3 mm contains most
lateral canals and deltas. This is
removed by resection

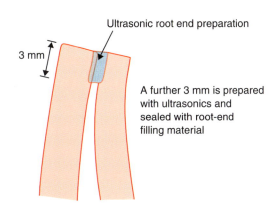

Ultrasonic root end preparation

A further 3 mm is prepared
with ultrasonics and
sealed with root-end
filling material

**Figure 10.7**

Root end preparation.

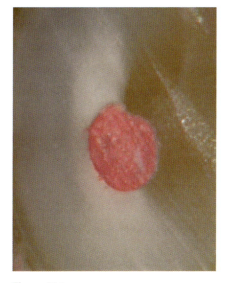

**Figure 10.8**

The root end has been smoothed with a tungsten carbide
bur prior to root end cavity preparation.

It is possible to use a 1% solution of
methylene blue dye to indicate the periodontal
ligament and help increase visibility of the
resected root tip. The dye is placed into the
bony crypt for approximately 10 seconds with
a sponge applicator. Ideally, cotton wool
should not be used during root end surgery as
cotton fibres have been shown to induce
foreign body reaction in the tissues. Methylene

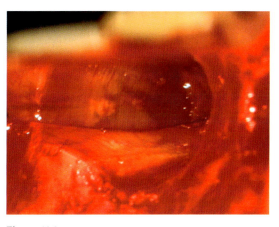

**Figure 10.9**

The resected root end of a maxillary first molar. Gutta
percha is visible in two separate canals. The canals are
joined by an isthmus. This detail would only be visible
under microscopic magnification and illumination.

blue dye will also highlight the presence of
any interconnections between canals or isthmi
and the presence of root fractures.

## Root End Preparation

Root end preparation is normally carried
out under the operating microscope using
ultrasonic instruments. There are micromirrors

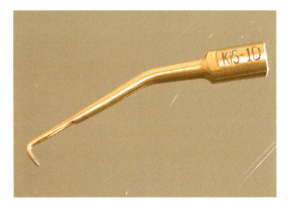

**Figure 10.10**

A KiS ultrasonic tip for root end cavity preparation. The tip has a diamond-coated end and an irrigant channel.

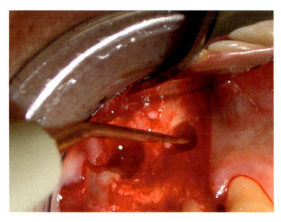

**Figure 10.11**

Preparation of a root end cavity in a maxillary premolar using a tip ultrasonic KiS.

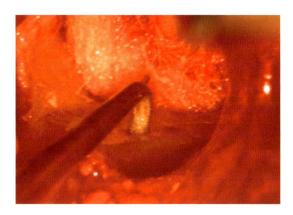

**Figure 10.12**

A high-magnification view of the ultrasonic tip being used to prepare the mesiobuccal root of a maxillary molar.

specifically designed for this. Stainless steel micromirrors come in different shapes and must be sterilized very carefully to avoid scratching on the surface. Alternatively, sapphire glass micromirrors are available. Specialist ultrasonic tips are angled to provide easy access to the resected root end. Many have irrigant channels to remove dentine chips as they are created and abrasive tips to improve cutting efficiency (Figure 10.10).

Generally, root end preparation is carried out to a depth of 2–4 mm.[5,6] In order to achieve an adequate seal the required depth will depend on the angle of bevel.[11] An increased bevel requires a greater length of preparation to prevent leakage of irritants through exposed dentinal tubules. The preparation is angled along the long axis of the tooth and the lateral borders will be dictated by the cross-sectional root canal anatomy following resection. While viewing the resected root end with an operating microscope, an ultrasonic tip can be guided along the root canal space to prepare and enlarge it. Ultrasonic tips are effective at debriding and enlarging canal anastomoses[6] and they achieve better shape and cleaner root end preparation compared with burs.[16,17] Care must be taken when using the ultrasonic tips without irrigant in confined or restricted access situations, as they can become very hot and there is a risk of burning the lip. After root end

preparation, the cavity is cleaned with sterile saline and then dried with a Stropko irrigator. Some studies have advocated the use of a conditioner such as citric acid to remove the smear layer. However, this may actually increase the amount of leakage.[18] Following drying, the cavity is inspected under higher magnification to ensure that all contours have been cleaned and shaped and that no lateral canals or anomalies have been missed (Figures 10.11–10.13).

## Root End Filling

In the majority of cases, root end surgery would not be carried out unless the root canal had been thoroughly cleaned prior to treatment. Therefore, in some cases it is not always necessary to prepare a retrograde cavity. In this situation, the gutta percha is burnished following resection of the root tip (Figures 10.14–10.16).

In order to place a root end filling, haemostasis must first be achieved.[19,20] Using an adequate quantity of local anaesthetic with

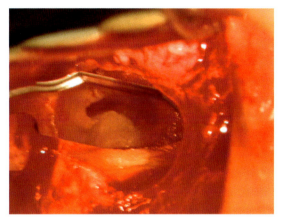

**Figure 10.13**

The completed root end preparation in the mesiobuccal root showing an isthmus between the root canals.

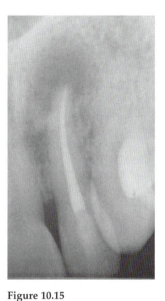

**Figure 10.15**

The root tip was resected. It was not considered necessary to place a root end filling as the case had only recently been retreated. The exposed gutta percha was burnished following root end resection.

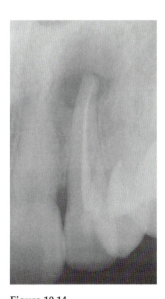

**Figure 10.14**

Root canal retreatment was recently completed in this maxillary lateral incisor but unfortunately symptoms did not resolve. Root end surgery was required.

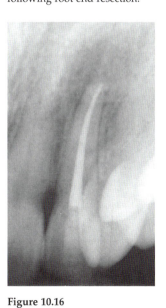

**Figure 10.16**

A review at 1 year showed good evidence of bony healing.

a vasoconstrictor is important, as is ensuring that the relieving incisions for flaps are made as vertical as possible. Horizontal incisions have the potential to cause more bleeding. A well-trained assistant using a microaspiration tip will help control small localized bleeds. Placement of haemostatic agents within the bony crypt will help control bleeding. Agents for use in endodontic surgery include the following.

### Gauze and Adrenaline (Epinephrine) Solutions

Pure surgical gauze that is fabricated from non-cotton fibres (and therefore less likely to initiate postoperative inflammation) can be dampened with 1:1000 adrenaline. The gauze is packed into the bony cavity for approximately 1 minute. Care must be taken with solutions containing high concentrations of adrenaline, especially in patients whose medical status may make them more sensitive. An alternative is to pack the gauze firmly into the bony crypt and then inject local anaesthetic containing 1:80 000 adrenaline into it. Haemostasis should be achieved within a few minutes.

### Gelfoam

Gelfoam (Pfizer Inc., New York, USA) is a gelatinous sponge-like material that expands on contact with blood and promotes the disintegration of platelets. Small pieces can be packed into the bony crypt to achieve haemostasis and do not necessarily need to be removed.[21]

### Surgicel

On contact with blood, Surgicel (Johnson & Johnson, New Brunswick, NJ, USA), which is a cellulose-based material, encourages the formation of a clot. It has been recommended that the material is removed following root end filling as it is not resorbable and may initiate a foreign body inflammatory response.[21,22]

### Ferric Sulphate

Concentrated ferric sulphate solution causes agglutination of blood proteins on contact. This in turn results in plugging of capillaries.

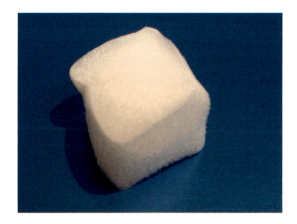

**Figure 10.17**

A collagen-based haemostatic agent can be placed in the bony crypt prior to placement of a root end filling.

The solution should be used sparingly, however, as it has been associated with postoperative difficulties.[23] The bony crypt should be curetted and washed out following the use of ferric sulphate solutions in order to remove remnants of the material and encourage fresh bleeding before flap closure.

### Collagen-Based Products

Hémocollagène (Spécialitiés-Septodont, Saint Maurdes-Fossés, France) and CollaCote (Colla-Tec Inc., Plainsborough, NJ, USA) are lyophilized collagen-based materials. Resorbable collagen-based agents can be left in the bony crypt and should not cause interference with healing (Figure 10.17).[15]

## Root-End Filling Materials

Virtually every conceivable restorative material has been utilized at some time as a root-end filling material. It is well documented that amalgam is no longer considered an appropriate material for use as a root end filling. It can be difficult to handle and it is not uncommon to see particles of amalgam alloy in the tissues surrounding the root end. Amalgam is prone to corrosion. Disintegration and release of metal particles into the surrounding tissue and gingivae can result in an amalgam tattoo. Mercury is toxic and its use may be a concern to patients. Since there are much more bio-compatible alternatives to amalgam, its use cannot be condoned. The healing characteristics following root end filling with amalgam are questionable and currently recommended materials all provide a superior seal.

From a biological and clinical perspective, there is good evidence for the use of the following materials in modern endodontic practice.

## Mineral Trioxide Aggregate

Mineral trioxide aggregate (MTA) is a powder consisting of fine hydrophilic particles. The chemical composition is similar to Portland cement, but without any impurities. Hydration of the MTA results in a wet, sand-like consistency that solidifies as it sets. The material has a long setting time (2 hours 45 minutes), which may be the reason for its superior sealing ability.[24,25] MTA is moisture tolerant and will set in the presence of moisture.[26] The material has shown excellent biocompatibility.[27] It is one of the few materials that has demonstrated cementum formation across its surface.[28] It can be technically demanding to employ MTA in root end surgery. MTA is loaded into the root end cavity in a carrier and plugged into place with micropluggers. The Lee block can be a useful device for loading MTA onto a flat plastic or plugger. Excess material is removed using a periodontal curette and the filling finished with a damp sponge. Due to the long setting time, no further refinement of the resected root end can be carried out. An alternative MTA material has been produced that has improved handling characteristics and contains added gypsum to decrease the setting time. A recent study has shown a high success rate with MTA as a root-end filling material. However, it had no significant advantage when compared with intermediate restorative material (IRM) (Figures 10.18–10.25).[29]

## Intermediate Restorative Material

Reinforced zinc oxide–eugenol cement such as IRM has been advocated as a root-end filling

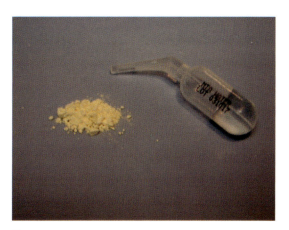

**Figure 10.18**

Mineral trioxide aggregate (MTA) is dispensed as a powder and water. When the two are mixed, the material takes on the consistency of wet sand.

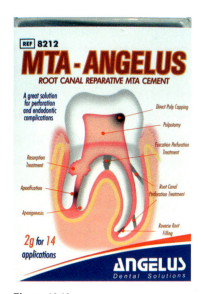

**Figure 10.19**

Modified MTA, with a faster setting time, may prove easier to manage.

material for many years. IRM can be placed into the root end cavity with a carrier or fine flat plastic and packed into place with micropluggers. The material is burnished against the root surface and, when set, the resected root end is finished with an ultrafine diamond or tungsten carbide bur, leaving a highly polished surface. This material produces a better seal than amalgam and periapical

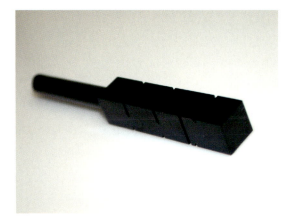

**Figure 10.20**

The Lee block is a device for creating small cubes of MTA that can be loaded onto a plugger or flat plastic.

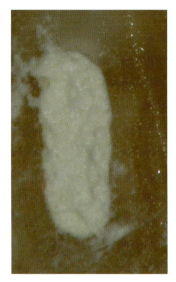

**Figure 10.22**

The cavity has been filled with ProRoot MTA and the surface wiped free of excess material with a damp sponge.

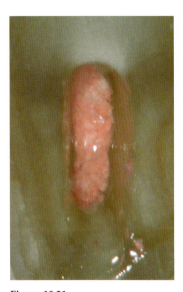

**Figure 10.21**

A view at high power showing the compacted gutta percha following root end cavity preparation.

healing following its use as a root-end filling material has generally been shown to be good (Figures 10.26–10.41).[30]

## Super EBA

Super EBA (ethoxybenzoic acid) is a modified zinc oxide–eugenol cement that has been

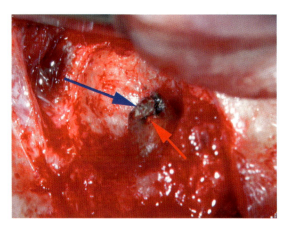

**Figure 10.23**

A previous attempt at root end surgery using amalgam as a root end filling can be seen in this maxillary central incisor (blue arrow). The case was retreated non-surgically to ensure that the root canal was adequately disinfected and the gutta percha root filling can be seen at the canal orifice (red arrow). The amalgam retrograde filling had been placed incorrectly and the root canal had not been prepared during surgery. It is perhaps not surprising that the previous attempt at endodontic surgery failed. The value of using an operating microscope is clearly highlighted.

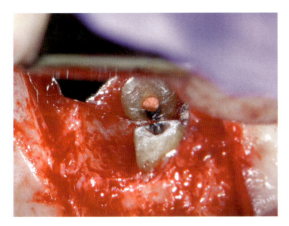

**Figure 10.24**

The amalgam filling was removed with ultrasonics and the root tip minimally resected to remove the bevel that had been made during previous surgery. An ultrasonic tip was used to prepare a root end cavity, and compacted gutta percha can be seen at the base of it.

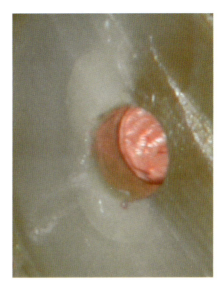

**Figure 10.26**

A view at high magnification following root end preparation with ultrasonics. The gutta percha is compacted with a microplugger as it becomes thermoplasticized by the ultrasonic tip.

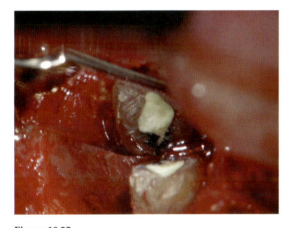

**Figure 10.25**

The case was filled with MTA. Because of the shortened root length it was not possible to remove all the stained dentine from the root tip without compromising the tooth. However, the root canal has been prepared and filled to a depth of 3–4 mm and should be well sealed.

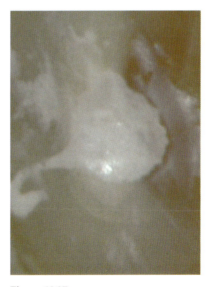

**Figure 10.27**

The root end cavity has been filled with IRM, which is burnished.

shown to have better sealing properties than amalgam and osseous repair following surgery.[31] The material is susceptible to moisture in the operative field and this may have a negative effect on the quality of seal.[26]

Microleakage was observed in root end cavities that were prepared ultrasonically and filled with Super EBA.[18] It has been recommended as a root end filling (Figures 10.42–10.44).

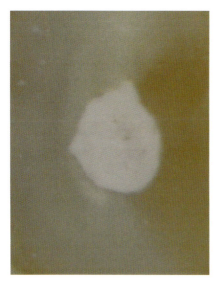

**Figure 10.28**

When the IRM has set, the resected root and filling material can be polished with an ultrafine diamond or tungsten carbide bur.

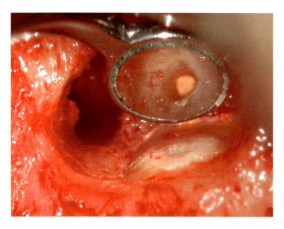

**Figure 10.29**

The completed root end preparation in a maxillary premolar.

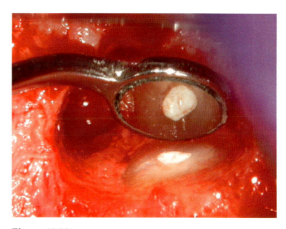

**Figure 10.30**

The case filled with IRM and the root surface polished.

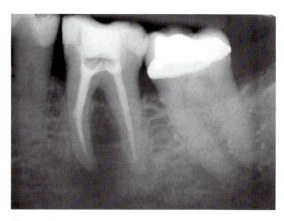

**Figure 10.31**

Non-surgical retreatment was completed on this mandibular molar. Unfortunately, there was a persistent buccal sinus tract which did not heal. Root end surgery was recommended.

## Glass Ionomer

There is a dynamic physicochemical bond between dentine and glass ionomer cement which enables the material to provide a seal when used as a root end filling. This sealing ability has been shown to be better than amalgam, and osseous healing adjacent to the material has been observed.[32] Glass ionomer can be placed across the entire resected root end, which is saucerized. This should also effectively seal exposed dentinal tubules. There are numerous clinical reports that support the use of glass ionomer.[33]

## Composite Resin

Dentine-bonded composite resin has been utilized as a root-end filling material, and in

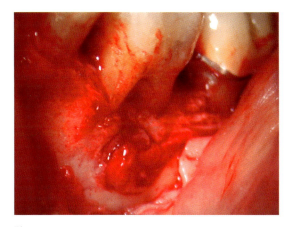

**Figure 10.32**

A triangular flap was raised to provide good surgical access.

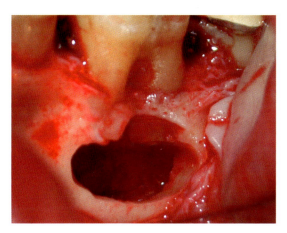

**Figure 10.33**

The lesion was curetted and the bony crypt enlarged to allow root resection and root end preparation of both roots.

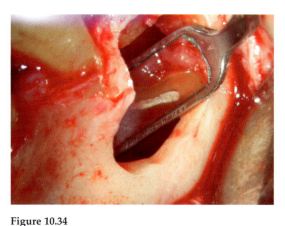

**Figure 10.34**

The completed root end filling in the mesial root, showing an isthmus connecting the two canals. This would not have been visible without an operating microscope.

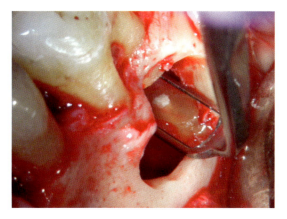

**Figure 10.35**

A view of the distal canal, showing the completed root end filling.

## Conditioning of the Resected Root End

the hands of skilled operators has shown promising results. Reformation of the periodontal apparatus and cementum has been reported adjacent to composite resin. The operating site must be moisture-free, which can be technically challenging. Therefore, placement of the material over the entire resected root end has been advocated. The material has superior sealing ability to amalgam.[34]

Some operators have recommended using an acidic conditioner on the resected root end to expose collagen fibrils and encourage healing. This method has been used following periodontal surgery to condition the root surface and stimulate reformation of the periodontal ligament.[35] In dogs, demineralization of the root end using citric acid has been shown to result in the predictable formation of new cementum.[36] Its effectiveness in humans has

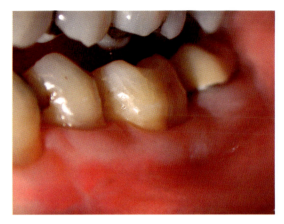

**Figure 10.36**

There was good healing by primary intention at the suture removal appointment 4 days following surgery.

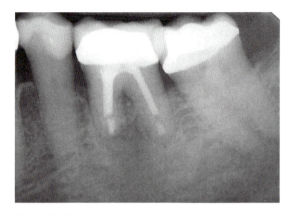

**Figure 10.38**

A review 1 year following treatment, showing complete bony healing.

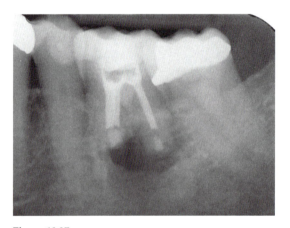

**Figure 10.37**

A radiograph of the case prior to replacement of the flap. There is at least 3 mm of root-end filling material in the root ends of both roots and the case should be well sealed.

not yet been ascertained, and this procedure may prove not to be necessary.[37]

## Radiographic Assessment

It is good practice to take a radiograph following placement of root-end filling material but prior to closure of the flap. This will allow the operator to make any adjustments or revision without risking the necessity of a second surgical procedure.

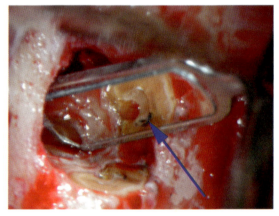

**Figure 10.39**

A maxillary first premolar with divergent roots. The case had been treated surgically on a previous occasion. Non-surgical retreatment had failed to relieve the patient's symptoms. Previous root end cavity preparation had missed the root canal, which was unprepared (blue arrow). The advantage of working with an operating microscope can clearly be appreciated.

The radiograph should show that:

- the root has been adequately resected and any remnants of the root tip completely removed
- the root-end filling material is well condensed and correctly adapted within the root end preparation
- there is no filling material or other foreign bodies scattered in the bony crypt.

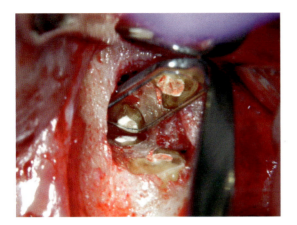

**Figure 10.40**

Both root ends were resected and root end cavities prepared with ultrasonics. They were filled with IRM.

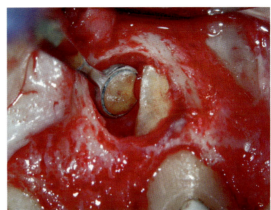

**Figure 10.42**

A maxillary incisor requiring root end surgery. Examination of the lateral aspect of the root with high magnification revealed a lateral orifice.

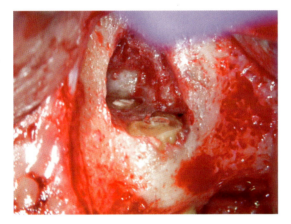

**Figure 10.41**

The root ends were polished with a tungsten carbide bur.

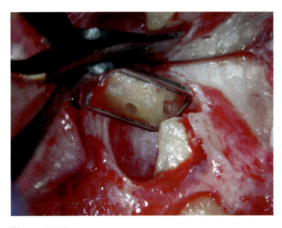

**Figure 10.43**

The root end has been resected and the apical and lateral orifices prepared with ultrasonics.

## REGENERATIVE PROCEDURES

Endodontic surgery has a much poorer prognosis when there has been loss of cortical bone overlying the root.[38] Regenerative procedures that are commonly used in periodontal surgery such as guided tissue regeneration (GTR) may be useful during endodontic surgery,[39] but there is currently little published evidence.

A classification of the situations in which GTR may be used in endodontic surgery is:[40]

- Class I: large periapical lesions without the involvement of the alveolar crest but where there has been significant destruction of the cortical plate or where both cortical plates have been perforated.[41]
- Class II: when a periapical lesion has direct communication to the alveolar crest – for example, when there has been loss of cortical plate, exposing the root surface and resulting in dehiscence.
- Class III: bone loss as a result of infection tracking along a developmental groove, furcal bone loss caused by perforation, defects resulting from cervical root resorption or oblique root fractures.

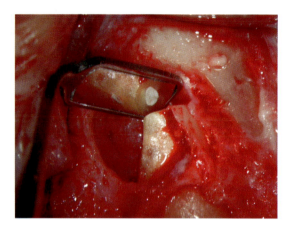

**Figure 10.44**

The case filled with Super EBA.

Membrane therapy was first introduced in 1969.[42] The membrane effectively separates bony healing from connective tissue healing. By delaying the advance of rapidly growing epithelial cells, the more slowly growing bone and periodontal ligament cells are encouraged to repopulate the root surface and produce new connective tissue attachments. The first membranes that were introduced were not absorbable and a second surgical procedure was required to recover the membrane following initial healing. Newer materials such as Bio-Gide are absorbable and tend to be preferred for this reason. Studies report that absorbable membranes appear to work effectively[43,44] and that the presence of the absorbable membrane has no deleterious effect on healing.

Following root resection and root end filling, the membrane is trimmed so that it covers the defect and rests on sound bone. The marginal border should be covered by gingiva when the flap is replaced.

## ROOT AMPUTATION AND HEMISECTION

Root amputation involves the removal of an individual root from a multi-rooted tooth, whereas hemisection results in complete sectioning of the tooth into separate halves.

Root amputation or hemisection may be considered in a well root-treated or retreated tooth in which the coronal portion of the root that is to be amputated has been filled with restorative material prior to surgery. Indications for surgery include:

- cases where there has been severe marginal periodontal disease around an entire root in a multi-rooted tooth, resulting in deep periodontal pocketing
- when there is caries preventing restoration of a root
- when iatrogenic difficulties such as perforation or previous apical surgery have resulted in a root becoming untreatable
- mesiodistal fracture of a maxillary molar
- buccolingual fracture of a mandibular molar.

### Case Selection

Usually, successful root amputation or hemisection can only be carried out in teeth where periodontal destruction has only affected one root and the treatment modality is beneficial to an overall treatment plan. The roots should be divergent and not fused and the furcation high. The prognosis is poor if there has been extensive bone loss around all the roots, the tooth is grade II or III mobile or the crown-to-root ratio is unfavourable.

### Root Amputation in Mandibular Molar

A flap is raised and any remaining bone removed over the root that is to be amputated. The root is sectioned from the furcation to the cement–enamel junction and elevated in a buccal direction. The resected surface should be smoothed, making sure there are no sharp retained spines of tooth. Following healing, the patient must be extremely vigilant in cleaning under the tooth to prevent caries.

### Hemisection of a Mandibular Molar

It is not always necessary to raise a flap for hemisection. The buccal and lingual grooves act as a guide for cutting. Traditionally, a silver cone was placed through the furcation to act as a guide. The occlusal surface is first reduced by 2–3 mm and then a high-speed bur with coolant water spray used to section the tooth. If one of the roots is to be removed, it can be elevated using luxators. Occasionally, the individual

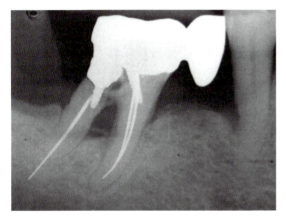

**Figure 10.45**

A failing root-filled tooth. There was evidence of marginal periodontitis, which required treatment. The distal root was fractured and unsaveable. The patient did not want a denture in the lower arch and was not a suitable candidate for implants. Hemisection of the molar was a possibility.

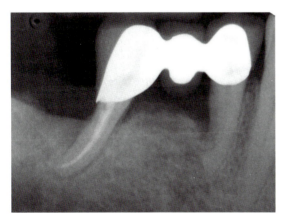

**Figure 10.46**

The mesial roots were retreated and the molar hemisected. A metal composite bridge has been constructed as a temporary measure. There appears to be good bony healing, and the teeth are not mobile. The patient is aware of the importance of good plaque removal around the bridge abutments.

roots can be restored as individual entities (bicuspidization). A radiograph is taken to confirm that there are no retained root fragments or foreign bodies and that there are no spurs or ledges associated with the retained root. The resected furcal surface is smoothed with a tungsten carbide or a diamond bur. The retained root will normally require restoration with a full-coverage crown (Figures 10.45, 10.46).

### Maxillary Teeth

One or both buccal roots can be amputated, as can the palatal root. Normally, a flap will be required to give adequate visibility and access. Maxillary molars can be hemisected in a mesiodistal direction (Figure 10.47).

## SURGICAL PERFORATION REPAIR

With the introduction of operating microscopes into endodontics, the methods available for repair of perforations using a non-surgical approach have increased enormously. However, there are occasions when a surgical approach may be required. Planning is very important, as access can be extremely difficult, especially if the root perforation is on the lingual surface.

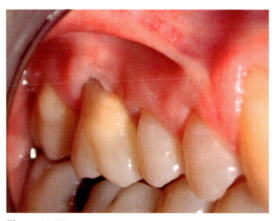

**Figure 10.47**

The mesiobuccal root of this maxillary molar has been resected. The patient has been instructed on oral hygiene measures to keep the area plaque-free.

Ironically, perforations occurring in the apical third pose least problems to surgical management. Generally, these are also easily managed using a non-surgical approach. Perforations made at the apex can be easily rectified with simple root end resection.

Normally, root canal retreatment will have been completed prior to surgical perforation repair. During this procedure, identification of the perforation site and an assessment of the likelihood of achieving access can be made. During surgery, the perforation site is located, cleaned and shaped using the ultrasonic tips that are used for root end preparation. The defect can then be sealed using root-end filling materials (Figure 10.48).

## POSTOPERATIVE INSTRUCTIONS

When surgery has been completed efficiently without unnecessary trauma to the surgical site, postoperative healing is usually uneventful. Patients should be provided with postoperative instructions both verbally and in writing. These will ensure good home care

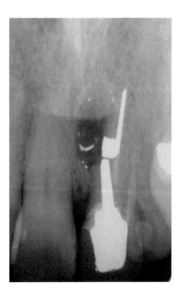

**Figure 10.48**

An attempt at surgical perforation repair has resulted in the demise of this tooth. The amalgam filling in the lateral aspect of the root does not seal effectively.

and improve both patient comfort and post-operative healing.

### Wound Care

- Eating and drinking is best avoided while the area is still numb, and the patient should have a soft diet until the sutures are removed, normally 3–7 days following surgery.
- Strenuous activity should be avoided for 24 hours.
- Alcohol and smoking should be avoided, as they will both have a deleterious effect on healing.
- The surgical site should not be disturbed for 24 hours. Consequently, the patient should be instructed not to pull the lip and try to avoid being overly inquisitive.
- Tooth-brushing can be omitted on the day of surgery, but recommenced the following day in all areas apart from the surgical site. The operative site is maintained using 0.2% chlorhexidine mouthwash. The solution is swilled for 1 minute twice daily. A saltwater rinse can be used after meals to help keep the area clean. A teaspoon of salt in a mug of warm water is sufficient.

### Postoperative Sequelae

#### Pain

Although there may be mild discomfort following root end surgery, severe pain is not usually a feature. The benefit of pre-emptive analgesia has already been discussed.

Postoperative pain can normally be controlled using non-steroidal anti-inflammatory drugs (NSAIDs) such as ibuprofen. Paracetamol or paracetamol and codeine is also effective for patients unable to use NSAIDs.[45,46] In order to measure the effectiveness of different medications two indicators are used:

- the percentage of patients that report over 50% pain relief in a 4–6 hour period compared with those receiving a placebo
- the number needed to treat (NNT).

The NNT is the number of patients that would need to be treated with a medicament as opposed to a placebo in order that one patient has a better outcome. The better the analgesic, the lower the NNT. This information can be obtained from the Pain Research Unit (Table 10.1).[47]

The most effective analgesic for reducing acute pain over 4–6 hours is 800 mg ibuprofen (NNT 1.6). Paracetamol 1000 mg combined with codiene 60 mg has an NNT of 2.2 and is the next best option should the patient be unable to take ibuprofen.

Combining paracetamol and NSAIDs has been shown to provide additive analgesia.[48] In a randomized, double-blind, placebo-controlled study, a combination of 600 mg ibuprofen and 1000 mg of paracetamol was significantly more effective in providing pain relief postoperatively following pulpectomy than 600 mg ibuprofen alone.[49] The results of this study suggest therefore that the combination of ibuprofen with paracetamol may be beneficial for postoperative endodontic pain relief. Combining paracetamol with codeine has also been shown to be an effective means of improving the therapeutic effect of paracetamol. In a randomized, double-blind, prospective trial, 1000 mg paracetamol with 30 mg codeine was significantly more effective in controlling pain for 12 hours following third molar removal than paracetamol alone.[50] Analgesics will be more effective if taken regularly, as this

will ensure that a therapeutic dose of drug is maintained in the bloodstream.

### Bleeding

Bleeding is unusual following surgery. However, the patient may taste blood in the mouth. Slight bleeding when mixed with saliva will always appear worse than it really is. Gently applying pressure to the operative site with a clean handkerchief or gauze for several minutes will usually alleviate the problem. If patients are concerned or there is significant bleeding, an emergency telephone number should have been made available for them to contact the surgeon.

### Swelling

Swelling may occur and is usually worse 24–48 hours following surgery. To reduce swelling, an icepack should be applied to the face for 20 minutes in each hour several times during the day of surgery.

### Bruising

Bruising can occur following surgery and is usually worse approximately 3–4 days following the procedure. It may take some time to resolve and can look rather alarming, even though it is completely painless (Figure 10.49).

**Table 10.1** *Analgesic efficacy*[a]

| Drug | Percentage > 50% relief | NNT[b] |
|------|-------------------------|--------|
| Ibuprofen 800 mg | 100 | 1.6 |
| Paracetamol 1000 mg and codeine 60 mg | 57 | 2.2 |
| Ibuprofen 600 mg | 79 | 2.4 |
| Ibuprofen 400 mg | 56 | 2.4 |
| Ibuprofen 200 mg | 45 | 2.7 |
| Paracetamol 500 mg | 61 | 3.5 |
| Paracetamol 1000 mg | 46 | 3.8 |
| Codiene 60 mg | 15 | 16.7 |
| Placebo | 18 | n/a |

[a] Information available from the Pain Research Unit, University of Oxford.

[b] The lower the number needed to treat (NNT), the more effective the drug.

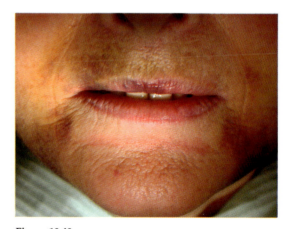

**Figure 10.49**

Bruising is possible following endodontic surgery.

## REVIEW FOLLOWING SURGERY

Within 2–3 days, an initial review appointment is required to remove any sutures and make an assessment of early healing. Further clinical and radiological examination is conducted at annual intervals until healing is observed.[51,52] Additional appointments may be required if complications arise.

Follow-up at 1 year is considered to be too short,[53,54] as there is likely to be bone formation at the periphery of the crypt following surgery irrespective of the status of the root tip. A period of 4 years is therefore considered to be a suitable benchmark.[55]

Healing can be classified into four headings (Figures 10.50, 10.51):[56]

- healed
- incomplete healing (scar)
- uncertain healing
- failed.

Incomplete healing with scarring is only considered stable after long-term follow-up. Some cases that may initially appear to have uncertain healing can sometimes improve. Equally, late failure (>10 years) has been reported in cases that appeared to be responding well,[57] although this study related to amalgam root end fillings.

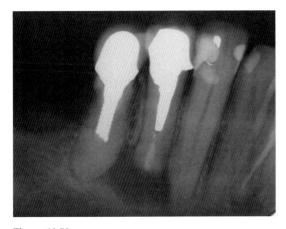

**Figure 10.50**

An MTA root end filling has been placed in the mandibular first premolar. Review would be undertaken at 1 year and then annually until healing occurred.

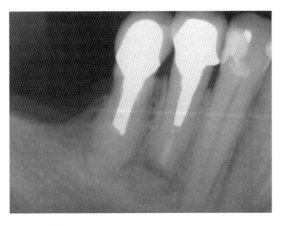

**Figure 10.51**

A review at 1 year shows good evidence of bony healing.

## REFERENCES

1. Gutmann JL. Principles of endodontic surgery for the general practitioner. *Dental Clinics of North America* 1984; **28:** 895–908.
2. Lin LM, Gagler P, Langeland K. Periradicular curettage. *International Endodontic Journal* 1996; **29:** 220–227.
3. Thompson IO, Phillips VM, Kalan M. Metastatic squamous carcinoma manifesting as a periapical lesion. *Journal of the Dental Association of South Africa* 1992; **47:** 481–483.
4. Byers M, Wheeler EF, Bothwell M. Altered expression of NGF and P75 NGF-receptor by fibroblasts of injured teeth precedes sensory nerve sprouting. *Growth Factors* 1992; **6:** 41–52.
5. Rud J, Andreasen JO. Operative procedures in periapical surgery with contemporaneous root filling. *International Journal of Oral Surgery* 1972; **1:** 297–310.
6. Kim S, Pecora G, Rubinstein RA. *Colour atlas of microsurgery in endodontics.* London: WB Saunders; 2001.
7. Chong BS, Pitt Ford TR, Kariyawasam SP. Tissue response to potential root-end filling materials in infected root canals. *International Endodontic Journal* 1997; **30:** 102–114.
8. Tidmarsh BG, Arrowsmith MG. Dentinal tubules at the root ends of apicected

teeth: a scanning electron microscopic study. *International Endodontic Journal* 1989; **22:** 184–189.

9. Carrigan PJ, Morse DR, Furst ML, Sinai IH. A scanning electron microscopic evaluation of human dentinal tubules according to age and location. *Journal of Endodontics* 1984; **10:** 359–363.

10. Ichesco WR, Ellison RL, Corcoran JF, Krause DC. A spectrophotometric analysis of dentinal leakage in the resected root. *Journal of Endodontics* 1991; **17:** 503–507.

11. Gilheany PA, Figdor D, Tyas MJ. Apical dentin permeability and microleakage associated with root end resection and retrograde filling. *Journal of Endodontics* 1994; **20:** 22–26.

12. Hsu YY, Kim S. The resected root surface. The issue of canal isthmuses. *Dental Clinics of North America* 1997; **41:** 529–540.

13. Wada M, Takase T, Nakanuma K, Arisue K, Nagahama F, Yamazaki M. Clinical study of refractory apical periodontitis treated by apicectomy. Part 1. Root canal morphology of resected apex. *International Endodontic Journal* 1998; **31:** 53–56.

14. Nedderman TA, Hartwell GR, Portell FR. A comparison of root surfaces following apical root resection with various burs: scanning electron microscope evaluation. *Journal of Endodontics* 1988; **14:** 423–427.

15. Gutmann JL, Harrison JW. *Surgical endodontics.* Cambridge: Blackwell; 1991.

16. Gutmann JL, Saunders WP, Nguyen L, Guo IY, Saunders EM. Ultrasonic root-end preparation. Part 1. SEM analysis. *International Endodontic Journal* 1994; **27:** 318–324.

17. Sultan M, Pitt Ford TR. Ultrasonic preparation and obturation of root-end cavities. *International Endodontic Journal* 1995; **28:** 231–238.

18. Saunders WP, Saunders EM, Gutmann JL. Ultrasonic root-end preparation. Part 2. Microleakage of EBA root-end fillings. *International Endodontic Journal* 1994; **27:** 325–329.

19. Witherspoon DE, Gutmann JL. Haemostasis in periradicular surgery. *International Endodontic Journal* 1996; **29:** 135–149.

20. Kim S, Rethnam S. Hemostasis in endodontic microsurgery. *Dental Clinics of North America* 1997; **41:** 499–511.

21. Olson RA, Roberts DL, Osbon DB. A comparative study of polyactic acid, Gelfoam and Surgicel in healing extraction sites. *Oral Surgery* 1982; **53:** 441–449.

22. Ibarrola JL, Bjorenson JE, Austin BP, Gerstein H. Osseous reactions to three haemostatic agents. *Journal of Endodontics* 1985; **11:** 75–93.

23. Jeansonne BG, Boggs WS, Lemon RR. Ferric sulfate hemostasis: effect on osseous wound healing. II. With curettage and irrigation. *Journal of Endodontics* 1983; **19:** 174–176.

24. Torabinejad M, Hong CU, Lee SJ, Monsef M, Pitt Ford TR. Investigation of mineral trioxide for root end fillings in dogs. *Journal of Endodontics* 1995; **21:** 603–608.

25. Torabinejad M, Wilder-Smith P, Kettering JD, Pitt Ford TR. Comparative investigation of marginal adaptation of mineral trioxide aggregate and other commonly used root-end filling materials. *Journal of Endodontics* 1995; **21:** 295–299.

26. Torabinejad M, Higa RK, McKendry DJ, Pitt Ford TR. Dye leakage of four root end filling materials: effects of blood contamination. *Journal of Endodontics* 1994; **20:** 159–163.

27. Chong BS. MTA-many tested applications. *Dentistry* 2001; **2:** 18–20.

28. Torabinejad M, Pitt Ford TR, McKendry DJ, Abedi HR, Miller DA, Kariyawasam SP. Histologic assessment of mineral trioxide aggregate when used as a root end filling in monkeys. *Journal of Endodontics* 1997; **23:** 225–228.

29. Chong BS, Pitt Ford TR, Hudson MB. A prospective clinical study of Mineral Trioxide Aggregate and IRM when used as root-end filling materials in endodontic surgery. *International Endodontic Journal* 2003; **36:** 520–526.

30. Pitt Ford TR, Andreasen JO, Dorn SO, Kariyawasam SP. Effect of IRM root end fillings on healing after replantation. *Journal of Endodontics* 1994; **20:** 381–385.

31. Pitt Ford TR, Andreasen JO, Dorn SO, Kariyawasam SP. Effect of Super EBA as a

root end filling on healing after replantation. *Journal of Endodontics* 1995; **21:** 13–15.

32. Pitt Ford TR, Roberts GJ. Tissue response to glass ionomer retrograde root fillings. *International Endodontic Journal* 1990; **23:** 233–238.

33. Chong BS, Pitt Ford TR, Watson TF. Light-cured glass ionomer as a retrograde root seal. *International Endodontic Journal* 1993; **26:** 218–224.

34. Rud J, Andreasen JO, Rud V. [Retrograde root filling utilizing resin and dentine bonding agent: frequency of healing when compared to retrograde amalgam]. *Danish Dental Journal* 1989; **93:** 267–273. [in Danish]

35. Crigger M, Renvert S, Bogle G. The effect of topical citric acid application on surgically exposed periodontal attachment. *Journal of Periodontal Research.* 1983; **18:** 303–305.

36. Craig KR, Harrison JW. Wound healing following demineralization of resected root ends in periradicular surgery. *Journal of Endodontics* 1983; **19:** 339–347.

37. Meyers JP, Gutmann JL. Histological healing following surgical endodontics and its implications in case assessment: a case report. *International Endodontic Journal* 1994; **27:** 339–342.

38. Skoglund A, Persson G. A follow-up study of apicoectomized teeth with total bone loss of the buccal bone plate. *Oral Surgery, Oral Medicine, Oral Pathology* 1985; **59:** 78–81.

39. Rankow HJ, Krasner PR. Endodontic applications of guided tissue regeneration in endodontic surgery. *Journal of Endodontics* 1996; **22:** 34–43.

40. von Arx T, Cochran DL. Rationale for the application of the GTR principle using a barrier membrane in endodontic surgery: a proposal of classification and literature review. *International Journal of Periodontics and Restorative Dentistry* 2001; **21:** 127–139.

41. Pecora G, Kim S, Celletti R, Davarpanah M. The guided tissue regeneration principle in endodontic surgery: one year postoperative results of large periapical lesions. *International Endodontic Journal* 1995; **28:** 41–46.

42. Boyne PJ. Restoration of osseous defects in maxillofacial casualties. *Journal of the American Dental Association* 1969; **78:** 767–776.

43. Caffesse RG, Mota LF, Quinones CR, Morrison EC. Clinical comparison of resorbable and non-resorbable barriers for guided periodontal tissue regeneration. *Journal of Clinical Periodontology* 1997; **24:** 747–752.

44. Camelo M, Nevins ML, Lynch SE, Schenk RK, Simion M, Nevins M. Periodontal regeneration with an autogenous bone-Bio-Oss composite graft and a Bio-Gide membrane. *International Journal of Periodontics and Restorative Dentistry* 2001; **21:** 109–119.

45. Mehlisch DR, Sollecito WA, Helfrick JF, Leibold DG, Markowitz R, Schow CE, Shultz R, Waite DE. Multicenter clinical trial of ibuprofen and acetaminophen in the treatment of postoperative dental pain. *Journal of the American Dental Association* 1990; **121:** 257–263.

46. Seymour RA, Ward-Booth P, Kelly PJ. Evaluation of different doses of soluble ibuprofen and ibuprofen tablets in postoperative dental pain. *British Journal of Oral and Maxillofacial Surgery* 1996; **34:** 110–114.

47. Pain Research Unit http://www.jr2.ox.ac.uk

48. Breivik E, Barkvoll P, Skovlund E. Combining diclofenac with acetaminophen or acetaminophen-codeine after oral surgery: a randomized, double-blind, single-dose study. *Clinical Pharmacology and Therapeutics* 2000; **66:** 625–635.

49. Menhinick KA, Gutmann JL, Regan JD, Taylor SE, Buschang PH. The efficacy of pain control following nonsurgical root canal treatment using ibuprofen or a combination of ibuprofen and acetaminophen in a randomized, double-blind, placebo-controlled study. *International Endodontic Journal* 2004; **37:** 531–541.

50. Macleod AG, Ashford B, Voltz M, Williams B, Cramond T, Gorta L, Simpson JM. Paracetamol versus paracetamol-codeine in the treatment of post-operative dental pain: a randomized, double-blind, prospective trial. *Australian Dental Journal* 2002; **47:** 147–151.

51. Halse A, Molven O, Grung B. Follow-up after periapical surgery: the value of the one-year control. *Endodontics and Dental Traumatology* 1991; **7:** 246–250.

52. Worrall SF. Are postoperative review appointments necessary following uncomplicated minor oral surgery? *British Journal of Oral and Maxillofacial Surgery* 1996; **34:** 495–499.

53. Grung B, Molven O, Halse A. Periapical surgery in a Norwegian county hospital: follow-up findings of 477 teeth. *Journal of Endodontics* 1990; **16:** 411–417.

54. Rud J, Andreasen JO, Jensen JE. A follow-up study of 1,000 cases treated by endodontic surgery. *International Journal of Oral Surgery* 1972; **1:** 215–218.

55. Rud J, Andreasen JO, Jensen JE. Radiographic criteria for the assessment of healing after endodontic surgery. *International Journal of Oral Surgery* 1972; **1:** 195–214.

56. Molven O, Halse A, Grung B. Observer strategy and the radiographic classification of healing after endodontic surgery. *International Journal of Oral and Maxillofacial Surgery* 1987; **16:** 432–439.

57. Frank Al, Glick DH, Patterson SS, Weine FS. Long-term evaluation of surgically placed amalgam fillings. *Journal of Endodontics* 1996; **18:** 391–398.

# INDEX

Page numbers referring to tables and figures are highlighted in **bold** and *italics* respectively.